DIRTY, LAZY, KETO®

Also by Stephanie Laska

The DIRTY, LAZY, KETO Cookbook:
Bend the Rules to Lose the Weight!

The DIRTY, LAZY, KETO Dirt Cheap Cookbook

DIRTY, LAZY, KETO Fast Food Guide:
Ten Carbs or Less

DIRTY, LAZY, KETO®

GET STARTED LOSING WEIGHT
WHILE BREAKING THE RULES

STEPHANIE LASKA

ST. MARTIN'S
ESSENTIALS
NEW YORK

First published in the United States by St. Martin's Essentials, an imprint of St. Martin's Publishing Group.

DIRTY, LAZY, KETO. Copyright © 2020 by Stephanie Laska. Foreword copyright © 2020 by Michael W. Jones. All rights reserved. Printed in the United States of America. For information, address St. Martin's Publishing Group, 120 Broadway, New York, NY 10271.

www.stmartins.com

The Library of Congress Cataloging-in-Publication Data is available upon request.

ISBN 978-1-250-62109-2 (trade paperback)
ISBN 978-1-250-62190-0 (ebook)

Our books may be purchased in bulk for promotional, educational, or business use. Please contact your local bookseller or the Macmillan Corporate and Premium Sales Department at 1-800-221-7945, extension 5442, or by email at MacmillanSpecialMarkets@macmillan.com.

First Edition: May 2020

10 9 8 7 6 5 4

I dedicate this book to the love of my life, Wild Bill. We ran, often stumbled, but lived every step in this journey together. I couldn't have done any of this without you as my partner.

To Charlotte and Alex, thank you for being patient with your mom. I know it's been a sacrifice.

CONTENTS

FOREWORD

Throughout the history of modern medicine, suspicion has been sporadically raised that perhaps obesity is more complex than we have ever understood. This was specifically noted by the editors in a 1924 issue of the *Journal of the American Medical Association*.* In 2013 this same AMA finally revised its long-held stance—or perhaps I should say *lack* of a stance—when it recognized obesity as a distinct disease state in its own right.† Why, you might ask, did it take so long? While there have been glimmers of the complexity of this recognition for quite some time, medical science has only in the last couple of decades begun to accumulate a critical mass of evidence to make this more definitively convincing. Not only has our new and rapidly growing under-

---

* "What Causes Obesity?" *Journal of the American Medical Association* 83, no. 13 (1924): 1003.
† Andrew Pollack, "A.M.A. Recognizes Obesity as a Disease," June 18, 2013, accessed March 13, 2019, http://www.nytimes.com/2013/06/19/business/ama-recognizes-obesity-as-a -disease.html

standing confirmed that obesity is a disease, but that it is, in fact—much like diabetes, heart disease, and other illnesses—a *chronic* disease that requires aggressive, life-long treatment. One of the take-home messages here: OBESITY is not a dirty word; it is a clinical condition, and its treatment should not be considered optional, but essential. Let's call it what it is and attack it aggressively.

What does this treatment look like? It may be a surprise to many that fifty-eight distinct causes of obesity have now been identified. This being the case, it should be no surprise, then, that there is no one-size-fits-all treatment. In fact, in my experience, one size often does not even fit one permanently. It is frequently necessary to tweak or even radically change treatment strategies throughout the "journey." If applied judiciously, current obesity treatment options include, and sometimes will require, the use of prescription medications as well as bariatric surgical interventions. As a brief aside, you should be aware that medications and surgery are NOT easy ways out. All the same, long-term treatments must be employed, or weight regain is quite likely; by current data, about 85 percent likely in two years or less. However, it should ALWAYS and forevermore include appropriate dietary and lifestyle modifications. While, for a particular individual, this may or may not turn you into the healthiest YOU that you can be, one thing is certain: without it, you will not achieve improved health. Dietary and lifestyle changes MUST be the foundation of any successful treatment, though *how* these are implemented often varies from person to person.

You may also be interested to know that there are currently no over-the-counter "weight-loss" supplements that have been shown any more effective than placebos in randomized controlled trials.* In addition, as far back as 2010, the Obesity Medicine Association has issued a position statement opposing the use of HCG (human chorionic gonadotropin, a hormone whose production is increased in women during pregnancy and for many years has been used in some, less reputable, weight-loss centers for its supposed benefit) in the treatment of obesity based on solid evidence of its utter lack of efficacy.† Please do not waste your money!

If diet is a critical link in the chain of obesity treatment, which diet should you use? As you might expect me to say, this varies. *Food is medicine.* I didn't make this up. Hippocrates, the Father of Medicine, in the early fourth century BC is said to have admonished patients to "Let food be thy medicine." To a fair extent, the "chemistry" of different foods will affect different individuals in various ways and help control their obesity to varying extents.

As this is a foreword to Stephanie Laska's *DIRTY, LAZY, KETO,* I feel it appropriate to put a non-shameless plug in for the ketogenic-type diet. While this diet strategy has reached "fad" status in our day and is plastered all over the internet and social media, it has been used medicinally for quite some time. In the United States and beyond, as far back as the 1920s, it began to be used relatively successfully in the treatment of childhood epilepsy. We also have reason to believe

---

* Joint Position Statement of Obesity Action Coalition, Obesity Medicine Association (formerly the American Society of Bariatric Physicians), Academy of Nutrition and Dietetics, October 2015.
† Position Statement: "Use of HCG in the Treatment of Obesity," Obesity Medicine Association, November 2010.

that Hippocrates himself treated some conditions with dietary restrictions that would have ostensibly been ketogenic. Unfortunately, despite the term becoming well-known, what has not become nearly as well understood is what it actually is and why it can be helpful. In many of my patients, "keto" has been confused with the Atkins Diet. Other than both diet types striving for very low carbohydrate intake, they are quite different.

The Atkins Diet, in addition to being a very low-carb regimen, strives for high-protein and moderate-fat intake. Keto is the reverse: *moderate protein* and *high fat*. You read that correctly—high fat! Obviously, leaning more toward the healthier (unsaturated) fats is preferable, but saturated fats are generally not off-limits. Why is this potentially beneficial for weight loss? Without getting too "scientific" (to use Stephanie's term), much of our production of fat is induced by sugar intake. In short, glucose (sugar breaks down into glucose) stimulates insulin production in the pancreas. Insulin signals the fat cells to make new fat and prevents the breakdown of fat to be used for energy. So more sugar intake = more fat-making and less fat-burning. So why only *moderate* protein intake? Protein is generally good, however if we take in too much, our cells can convert amino acids (the building blocks of proteins) into sugar. In addition, high-protein intake over time can, in some situations, overtax the kidneys. For keto, the bottom line is this: if we effectively "starve" our cells of sugar, they will have to begin using more fat as a source of fuel rather than storing it. The term "ketogenic" simply comes from the fact that a by-product of our cells utilizing fat is the production of "ketones." More and more we are discovering why some are calling ketones "brain food," but that's for another discussion.

I have seen many individuals make good and effective use of a ketogenic diet, though of course it has not been equally effective for all. I think there are several reasons for this, some of which we just do not yet know; remember, the science undergirding our modern understanding of obesity remains in its relative infancy. However, some evidence and experiences help inform us as to the characteristics of the keto diet's degrees of both success and failure. Perhaps one of the most obvious reasons for failure is one's inability to adhere to the dietary restrictions. But why? Please do not beat yourself up about not having "enough willpower." **Obesity is not a willpower disease.** That is not to say willpower is not important, but, truthfully, no one has enough willpower to overcome this disease. An analogy I like is to compare willpower to the solid rocket boosters on the space shuttle. The boosters' fuel source is essential in what NASA calls "primary propulsion." In other words, the shuttle will not achieve liftoff and get in the air without it; however, it is completely insufficient at the task of settling the craft into orbit; this requires things like thrusters and gravity. The point being, while obesity is NOT a willpower problem, this does not mean that willpower is not helpful and even necessary, especially in the short term and perhaps in recurrent bursts. Over the long term we find we do not need inexhaustible willpower; rather we need hormone power: we need to change obesity from the inside out.

This, then, brings us to the question, Why DIRTY, LAZY, KETO? Certainly, for many, adhering to a strict keto plan is indeed effective, but it can become progressively more onerous for some and they can lose "primary propulsion" before they are even close to settling into orbit, to extend our previous analogy. **What I have found in those patients for whom I have recommended DIRTY, LAZY, KETO is that, for many, it has simply been more *doable*.** It serves to relax the restrictions modestly but not to an extent that will tend to sabotage the metabolic and physiologic benefits of your dietary modification. Over the years I have rejected many of the attempts to make keto *easier*. Not because I do not like easier, but because often I find folks effectively avoiding the necessary "sugar starvation," which hijacks their ability to convert to fat metabolism to any helpful degree. I have not generally found that to be the case with DIRTY, LAZY, KETO.

Many have, and I suspect many more will, use DIRTY, LAZY, KETO as an integral and very effective part of their obesity treatment from start to finish. However, there are two other ways I use it with my patients. I work with some individuals who are responding very nicely to "regular" keto but who begin, for various reasons, to struggle. I will advise them to use DIRTY, LAZY, KETO to sort of give them a break for a time without sabotaging their progress. For others, even the thought of such a radical dietary change sends them nearly into paroxysms of panic. Some of these patients feel inspired by *DIRTY, LAZY, KETO* because the author is a *regular* person explaining it to regular people, removing the fear and leading to greater success. Some of these people go on to use this as a stepping stone to even more aggressive treatment.

Finally, I would be remiss if I closed without mentioning the respect I have gained for Stephanie. She is not a clinical person and is the first to disclaim this—however, I can tell you that she has done her homework. Some of that has obviously been through research and asking the right questions. Much of it has been through her own tireless struggle to feel better, live better, and live more. As extraordinary as her results may seem, I can tell you her accomplishments are not. Having worked with many people struggling with this disease, improved health is not just for those who write the books. You **can** do this! Stephanie and I wish you all the best in your journey.

—Dr. Michael W. Jones, DO, MBA, FAAFP
Medical Bariatrician, Lynchburg, Virginia

BACKGROUND

When I created DIRTY, LAZY, KETO, the only friend I had to ask for dieting advice was an alcoholic, Xanax-fueled friend with an eating disorder. That being said, I didn't have much guidance! I was lost and had no one to talk to. I didn't even know this way of life existed.

What I *did know* is that I was severely overweight— medically categorized as "severe" or "extreme" obesity, to be exact. I weighed close to 300 pounds. Even though (at the time) I didn't suffer from any obvious or immediate health problems, I knew if I didn't "do something," I would likely end up with type 2 diabetes, or worse, on an operating table having my stomach morphed into a ridiculous and unnatural shape. The fear of insulin shots or surgery (and fear of giving up Diet Coke—isn't that a requirement of bariatric surgery?) motivated me to consider all available options. **So how did I end up losing 140 pounds, about half of my total body weight?**

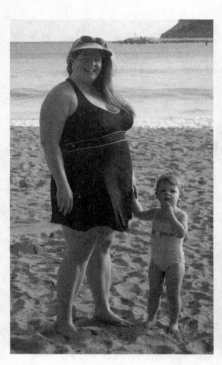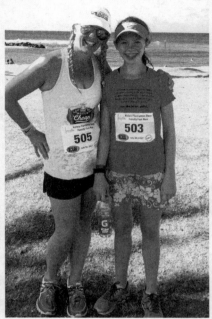

My pill-popping, wine-swilling friend got me started down the fateful path I would later groom into my current DIRTY, LAZY, KETO lifestyle. The purpose of this book is not to relive my entire journey, but rather to get you started exactly where I finished. Why should you waste time in your journey making the same mistakes that I did? You don't want to hear all that drama (or do you?). Oh, dear reader, if you are interested in all of THOSE details, then we are going to become lifelong friends!

Before we move forward, I bet you want to clear up a couple of things. . . .

WHAT DID YOUR FRIEND SAY? Now keep in mind

that what she told me is not the secret behind DIRTY, LAZY, KETO. The sea did not part, and lights from heaven did not shine down upon me; there was not even a chorus of angels singing "*Hallelujah!*" Quite the opposite: Our passing conversation was just the spark that ignited my motivation. Have you heard the saying "When the student is ready, the teacher shall appear"? Well, my teacher appeared as a middle-aged woman with a drinking problem!

I am happy to share with you the sad truth of what actually got me started. It's not glamorous, and actually it's downright embarrassing, but here goes: My friend shared that her formerly overweight husband was able to lose forty pounds pretty quickly by eating a ton of grilled chicken while still drinking beer.

SERIOUSLY! I thought, *Losing weight*
while still drinking beer?
NOW THAT'S MY KIND OF DIET.

So there it is. My friend went on to tick off the benefits of the Atkins Diet. You might remember Dr. Atkins from the 1970s? Of course you know who I'm talking about. No self-respecting overweight individual in America hasn't tried FREAKING EVERYTHING, right? I believed the Atkins program was about eating a lot of bacon, losing weight, and maybe having a heart attack, but other than that, I was actually pretty clueless. My training thus far about losing weight was limited to the calorie-restriction model served up from years of attending Weight Watchers meetings* and listening to the rants from my ever-weight-conscious grandmother.

I did glean *some information* from this Atkins conversation, though, that I would later find extremely helpful when embarking on my weight-loss pilgrimage. Specifically, I learned that increasing protein and lowering carbohydrate intake would magically cause my metabolism to change and help me lose weight. I didn't really care about all of the science behind how this worked, as I was mainly focused on the weight-loss part of the story (while enjoying eating grilled chicken and drinking beer). That sounded like a win/win to me!

I took these kernels of truth from Atkins and ran with them, morphing the rules AS I SAW FIT. Thus, I began the very long journey to where I stand today. It took about a year and a half to lose 140 pounds (roughly 10 pounds a month), and I've kept it off for seven years now. Over this time, with much trial and error (LOTS of trial, LOTS of error), I've finally arrived at my own successful eating lifestyle that I have earned the right to call DIRTY, LAZY, KETO.

Keep in mind, **this is my own version of keto.** I'm not following some website or existing plan touted by celebrities. This is the Stephanie Laska version, folks! What I'm about to share may challenge or even surprise you. So before you become alarmed and are thinking of summoning the keto police, I'd like to state the obvious: this here is my book, and I get to call the shots!

For our last bit of housekeeping, I would like to state that there is the potential for keto jargon to be used differently

---

* No disrespect to Weight Watchers. Their program works for a lot of people, just not for me.

here than how you may have heard it used before. I may even introduce some new terms or (gasp!) use terms in a new way. This is my own version of dirty or lazy keto and even, "LAWD, help me!" my own version of the combined "dirty AND lazy" keto! *(Are those of you who are new to this keto business wondering what all this shouting is about? Well, keto followers splinter off to a variety of different paths and can sometimes be devout and EVANGELICAL about their beliefs. Therefore, I don't want semantics to prevent learning.)*

I want to be the helpful friend to you that I never had. I want to give it to you straight and speak from experience. I come from a place of love, so forgive me if I challenge your beliefs about food or get it wrong occasionally. Truth be told, I welcome your feedback and hope to learn from you, too. Life is a journey, my friend, not a destination. I'm here for the entire ride.

I recently read a book about a meth addict and his sponsor. The message I took away from this memoir was how healing mentorship can be. The author talked about how his becoming a sponsor to an addict in need not only helped him "pay it forward," but, surprisingly, helped calm his own mind. Perhaps that is my motivation here. I feel I have been given a gift with my weight loss, and now I have a compulsion to help you, my dear reader, with the most difficult problem you likely have ever faced.

My goal is not to just get you started, but also to help support you through all the ups and downs you will likely experience on your own weight-loss journey. Obviously, you've had a spurt of motivation (or curiosity to get this far), so let's capitalize on that and get you moving. No need to be long-winded here. I'm telling you it worked for me, and if you picked up this book, you must be a teensy-tiny-bit curious and maybe willing to give this a try.

Will there be a lot of talk about the biology of weight loss? *Um, no.* That sounds really boring, and plus, I'm not qualified. Although I am a former public-school teacher with a master's degree in education, I will not be giving any science lessons here today, folks. Let's leave that up to the self-proclaimed keto experts, *whoever they are*! I'm not here to convince you to eat keto: lazy, dirty, or otherwise. I just know this way of eating has given me incredible results. I will give you enough sound bites to ward off your critical mother-in-law or insensitive coworkers, but that's about it. DIRTY, LAZY, KETO is based largely on my own personal struggle to lose 140 pounds and keep the weight off for seven years. *Mic Drop!*

Ultimately, I want to provide you with real-life inspiration and practical tips to get started on a DIRTY, LAZY, KETO lifestyle. I want to tell you my story—what I eat, how I shop—and show you what's on my plate. My stories will help you, surprise you, and maybe even make you laugh. To prepare you fully for what lies ahead, I want to warn you about other emotions that might surface. I cried a lot while writing this story, and it wasn't just when I said goodbye to cookies. *Being overweight is painful.* While I didn't want to examine "that part" of my life, I realized I couldn't fully breathe until I shed light on the areas of my life that tormented me. I surprised even myself by learning how these memories continue to haunt my adult life. I don't think I'm alone in my experiences being obese or when trying to lose weight. I'm betting you can identify with parts of my story, too.

TALK DIRTY TO ME

For additional free support, find helpful resources at:

https://dirtylazyketo.com/
Podcast! Listen to the author directly on the Podcast
DIRTY, LAZY, Girl

Get involved in the DIRTY, LAZY, KETO community at these sites:

www.facebook.com/dirtylazyketo
www.pinterest.com/dirtylazyketo/
www.instagram.com/dirtylazyketo/
www.instagram.com/140lost/
www.bit.ly/DLKYouTube
www.twitter.com/140lost

Join other fans of the DIRTY, LAZY, KETO community by joining the FREE author-led Facebook support group

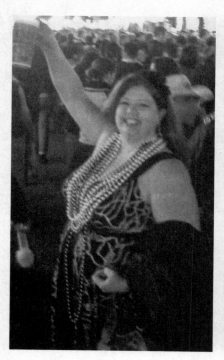
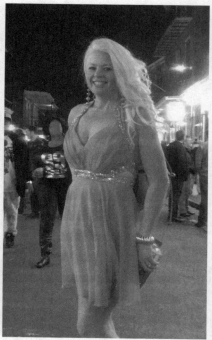

at www.facebook.com/groups/DirtyLazyKeto. If a smaller, more private, support group is preferred, I also host a more intimate, women only, limited enrollment, subscription-based premium group at https://www.facebook.com/groups/dirtylazyketopremium.

INTRODUCTION

The Police Will Never Find Me!

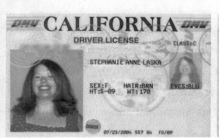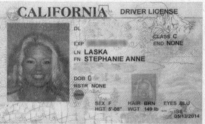

Since I have lived in a body that shrunk from size 26 to 4/6, I have earned the right to help you fight your obesity. I am not a nutritionist or a medical professional. I am just a regular wife and mother who has struggled with being overweight most of her life. I'm busy like you, and live paycheck to paycheck. I shop at Walmart and use coupons. Overall, I'm tired of trying to be perfect. I follow keto my own way, and from the look of my medical chart and pants size, my current lifestyle appears to be working!

What I lack in pedigree, I make up for with heart. My motivation is to help you, my dear reader, with the fight of your life. By the grace of God, I have been given some answers here, and I intend to shout these secrets from the rooftops. What I once thought of as a "metabolic miracle" has morphed into clarity.

**I didn't lose 140 pounds by accident.
I haven't kept that weight off for seven years due to
magic. I changed the way I ate and developed
new habits—plain and simple!**

Like an AA sponsor for carb addicts, I am proud to pass on what I have learned. I want you to replicate my results of healthy, sustainable weight loss. During this journey, I promise to speak to you as honestly as I would to my best friend. If my writing comes across as sassy, then I'm getting through loud and clear. DIRTY, LAZY, KETO isn't rocket science, and we don't need to overcomplicate this.

**Let me back up and properly introduce myself:
"Hi. My name is Stephanie and I'm a carboholic."**

I started this voyage wearing size 26 and weighing close to three hundred pounds. Even as a taller woman, according to the CDC* and the BMI (Body Mass Index) scale, I landed in the class 3 obesity category (which is the end of the line!).

---

* https://www.cdc.gov/obesity/adult/defining.html

In case you are not familiar with the dreaded BMI, let me give you the quick and dirty. BMI is a screening tool used to evaluate whether a body weight falls within a healthy range. BMI is calculated from an objective standardized math equation. A person's weight (in kilograms) is squared and then divided by their height (in meters). Complicated? *You betcha!* Whether or not this is an antiquated evaluation method for determining healthy weight is open for debate. Until it's changed, we are stuck with it! This screening tool is considered the standard of care in most doctor offices. So, unless you have a growth spurt or legitimately lose weight, there is no way to "game the system" and lower your BMI.

Speaking of height, I need to fess up to something quite embarrassing. For my entire adult life, I have lied about how tall I am. I added imaginary inches to every form I've ever filled out. From the doctor's office to the DMV, on paper I grew to a fictitious five feet nine (or even five feet ten inches!) tall. If my body was lying in a ditch somewhere as the victim of a serial killer, the police would never match my identity with my driver's license. Why would I lie about such a thing? Because the taller you are, the more you are "allowed" to weigh; In full disclosure, I didn't just fib about my height; back then I "adjusted" my weight, too. *Somehow* my license said the first digit started with a *100* instead of *200* when it came to my weight—*oops!*

It wasn't until I was flying to attend a work meeting that I realized my weight might be spiraling out of control. My plane was preparing for takeoff when I was shocked to discover that my seat belt wouldn't close. *My stomach was simply too big.* I tried shifting my weight, sucking in my gut, and even performed a modified squat to try and get that sucker to clasp, but I did not have any success. I was too embarrassed to ask a flight attendant for help. Mortified, I chose to hide from the problem. I laid my suit jacket over my lap to cover the unhooked seat belt and pretended to be asleep. My secret was safe.

You might think that embarrassing moment would be enough to scare me into changing my eating habits, but it did not. Like any card-carrying carboholic, I was in denial about my addiction to sugar. Months later at Disneyland, I was riding the Big Thunder Mountain Railroad roller coaster when it really hit home. My companion on the ride, my five-year-old son, almost flew out of the roller coaster coming down the first hill. Because I was so large, the pull-down bar stopped only at my stomach, leaving a huge gap between the safety bar and my little boy. I spent the entire ride absolutely terrified—not because of the intended thrills, but because I was petrified that my unrestrained son was going to fly out of the car. Talk about a wake-up call! Happiest place on earth? NOT! If I wasn't going to lose the weight for myself, I would absolutely do it to protect my child.

That roller-coaster incident was a slap across my face, snapping me out of denial. I decided then and there, among the fairy princesses to witness my proclamation, that I absolutely had to find a way to lose weight, *no matter what*. At that moment, I would've done anything, absolutely anything, to "fix" my situation. I even wrestled with the option of weight-loss surgery. Before making that call, however, I decided to try one last dietary intervention. Enter the ketogenic-inspired approach to losing weight, where I discovered, by accident, that eating higher fat, moderate-protein, low-carbohydrate foods would help me break the chains of obesity. With relatively quick success under my loosened belt, I felt hopeful for the first time in decades.

The traditional ketogenic diet, however, proved too confining for me. While I liked the overall concepts, the implementation, or "nitty-gritty," didn't seem realistic for my family. I couldn't understand how anyone could afford the ingredients, and I panicked whenever I was away from my own kitchen. The rules were too strict, but, more important, unsustainable. I quickly discovered that strict keto dieters give up everything fun: Artificial sweeteners like Splenda are frowned upon, so fat bombs and an innocent scoop of low-carb ice cream are out of the question, as is cold beer. *(Who invited THAT guy to the party?)*

Trying to eat "perfectly" all the time, I realized, would set me up for a lifetime of disappointment.

Who gives up Diet Coke and tortillas? Let's keep it real. My limited family budget didn't include organic vegetables, cage-free eggs, line-caught fish, or grass-fed butter. Call me crass, but at the time, most of my meals came from the microwave or a drive-thru. According to the keto books I read, that meant I was doomed to fail.

There had to be another way.

Instead of becoming a follower of the keto flock, I strayed. I morphed the diet's principles into a program that made sense to me. I kept what worked and discarded unnecessary rules. After much trial and error, I bucked the system by proving I could lose a significant amount of weight and keep it off *for years* (YEARS!). The only catch? I had to do it my way! The result was a kinder, more inclusive version of the low-carb, higher fat keto diet, which included sugar substitutes, grain alternatives, and a more flexible method of counting macro-nutrients. I discovered I could have my sugar-free cake and eat it, too. *Hallelujah!*

#BreakTheRules

Is losing weight really just about food? Definitely NOT! If it were that simple, we could throw the bread away and be done with it. Unfortunately, losing weight is not that simple. DIRTY, LAZY, KETO is more than just bacon and butter: *it's a lifestyle.*

WHAT IS
DIRTY, LAZY, KETO?

To put it simply, the keto lifestyle consists of eating foods higher in fat, moderate in protein, and lower in carbohydrates. When followed precisely, keto dieters calculate and adhere to macronutrient goals, like eating approximately 70 percent of their daily calories from fat, 25 percent from protein, and the remaining 5 percent of calories from carbohydrates. How these ratios translate into grams will vary according to how many calories per day a person actually eats.

Let's think about applying this to an actual person to see how this makes sense. Someone eating 2,000 calories per day would eat 1,400 calories just from fat. Since a fat gram has 9 calories, that equates to 156 grams of fat per day. To do this "correctly," many argue, every bite of food must be measured and accounted for. Ingredients should be "clean"—meaning of the highest quality. *There is no wiggle room!* Consistently following this regimen forces the body to burn fat, which leads to weight loss.

Easy-peasy, right? Not so fast. The keto diet, as you just read about, is pretty dang strict! There is a lot of stressful math, and to tell you an embarrassing secret, I had to pull out a calculator *like three times* (and take two Tylenols) trying to figure out all those numbers. Does it really need to be so complicated? I don't think so!

In my experience, I was able to lose weight by NOT eating clean and NOT stressing myself out with complex math. Call me a keto rebel, but I figured out a much easier way.

#BreakTheRules

DIRTY, LAZY, KETO is a way to lose weight without obsessing over calorie counting or buying fancy groceries.

The term "lazy" in keto-land means "to hell with all that extreme documentation of every morsel of food you pop in your mouth." Before you rush to any judgment, understand that lazy keto dieters can be just as successful as those who follow a strict regimen. Lazy keto doesn't mean dieters are relaxing in the shade somewhere.

**"Lazy" is just a coined term that describes a
way of focusing on *carb count only*
(not fat, protein, or calories).**

This is different from tracking. Lazy keto dieters *may or may not* document everything they eat (on paper or using an app), but they certainly keep a close eye on their daily net carbs intake. In general, lazy keto followers choose lower carb, higher fat foods to enjoy while staying "under" or "around" their carb goals or limits for the day.

What's all this "dirty" business about? Is there some X-rated version of keto out there in cyberspace? (Probably.) This is a fun book, but not THAT kind of fun. Dirty keto dieters like to Break The Rules now and again with ingredient choices.

Dirty keto equates to being open-minded about sugar and grain substitutes, which can make a recipe feel more "like what we are used to."

Lastly, I like to think "dirty keto" also mean a "no-holds-barred" approach to dieting. We like to Break The Rules every once in a while. Flexibility is a key differentiator, making it possible to follow the lifestyle over the long haul.

HOW Does This Actually Work?
In a Word—*Ketosis*

For all of the data-driven readers, I'd like to offer my take on why DIRTY, LAZY, KETO actually causes weight loss. Sharpen your pencils and get out your calculators—*kidding*! Now without going into a bunch of science (snooooooooooze . . .), I want to give you enough info here to ward off questions from any critical, or rude coworkers and family skeptics. If you want to skip all of this background, go for it. Knowing the scientific explanation behind ketosis isn't going to make your weight come off any faster. There are a lot of science experts out there who can help explain this a lot better than I can, I'll admit. But you know what they won't be able to tell you? . . . How this all works from a former fat girl's perspective. *Yup, I'm going there.* I'm going to rattle your ingrained beliefs about food.

When I lost my weight, I had no idea what was happening. In fact, I was pretty mystified by the whole thing! None of it made sense to me at the time. I was like a little kid seeing what I could get away with.

"Cheese? Ranch dressing?"

Sure, I'll eat that and see what happens. WOW. I still lost weight that week.

This is the WEIRDEST LIFESTYLE EVER! went through my mind every time I got on the scale and saw *continued weight loss* despite eating higher fat foods.

While I didn't want to ask too many questions (feeling like I would jinx the whole thing), I understand that you might be approaching this diet a bit more skeptically than I did. In fact, I learned all of this much later but am happy to share with you my armchair understanding of how it works.

The purpose of following a ketogenic diet is to burn fat. That sounds good, right? Who wants to be fat? But to lose weight, you have to *eat fat*? Now that part is confusing (and a bit ironic). When the body is fed a diet low in carbohydrates, moderate in protein, and higher in fats, a new metabolic state is induced called *ketosis*. Ketosis keeps the body running using fat. This is completely different from using carbs as an energy source—*glycolysis*. Did I lose you there? Me, too. You really don't need to know any of this, but I don't want you to be embarrassed when someone asks, "Why are you eating mayonnaise if you are on a diet?"

You can smartly reply, "Eating fat helps put my body in ketosis!"

Now you sound legit.

I am going to tell it to you straight. I lost 140 pounds on a low-carb diet without knowing what the word "ketosis" meant. From a medical standpoint, I had no clue what was happening "behind the scenes" that biologically caused my weight loss of roughly 10 pounds a month. When I finally looked up the term "ketosis," I was like, "HUH! So, *that's* why!"

Everyone tosses the word "ketosis" around in keto-land, though, so knowing what it means might be worth understanding.

"Ketosis" is just a fancy word that explains HOW the body is being fueled by FAT.

Like a fire, your body runs on fuel or it just fizzles out. There are only two natural energy sources available to fuel your fire: ketones (fat) or glucose (carbs).

Why is this important? If you feed your fire (body) too much of the wrong fuel (carbs), the excess is stored as fat. Consuming too much of the wrong fuel leads you to either GAIN WEIGHT or MAINTAIN an overweight body. On the flip side, if you cut back on the amount of this fuel you give your body, it looks elsewhere for a new supplier of fat—like from your ass! HA! Got your attention now, right? THAT'S KETOSIS, PEOPLE!

I don't know about you, but I like the sound of this ketosis business. Please, dear body, use my ass for all future energy sources.

How can you help your body go into ketosis? By eating a ketogenic diet rich in fats, moderate in protein, and low in carbohydrates, your body quickly burns through available glucose (from the carbs in the food you just ate) and then switches over to the "fat-burning" mode. That's how you lose weight. It's REALLY that simple. *Thank you, ketosis!*

How do you know when ketosis is happening? Please don't buy those weird pee strips. First of all, trying to pee on a piece of paper is kind of gross; but perhaps more important, it's unnecessary. A few magical things happen during ketosis that are a big 'ole giveaway: bad breath, increased urination, and weight loss. *This is true.*

Ketosis is the magical condition that helps me refrain from overeating and gaining weight (or maintaining an overweight body). Running my body on ketones also helps me only eat what my body actually needs. I automatically reduce my caloric intake (WITHOUT COUNTING CALORIES!). My energy levels and mood feel stabilized. I'm no longer searching in the kitchen or going through drive-thrus for food to help "lift me up." I feel normal for the first time in my life! This is how I lost weight, my friends. DIRTY, LAZY, KETO IS A METABOLIC MIRACLE!

I would like to acknowledge the irony here of eating more fat to prevent getting fat or staying fat. I understand that it is shocking new information to many readers. To this day, I have to fight my impulses to NOT dip my artichoke into full-fat mayo. *It just seems wrong.* I was brought up in the 1980s, when fat was blamed for almost everything, like obesity and heart disease.

I come from an era when SnackWell's cookies and Jazzercise were supposed to solve all of my weight problems.

I'm here to tell you, as living proof, that we have been literally fed the wrong information for our entire lives. Fat is not evil; fat is satiating! **When fat is removed from packaged foods, sugar is often added as a replacement and to improve taste. The remaining product is now high in carbohydrates and left stripped of its original nutritious value.** This is *so wrong* on *so many* levels. Eating foods that are high in carbohydrates causes your blood sugar to go haywire; just ask any diabetic.

Let me step back. Think of your body as a car. You need to fuel your car to drive, right? When you go to the gas station, there are several choices for fuel—but the options essentially boil down to a choice between economy or premium gas. Who knows what the difference is? Don't we all just pick the cheapest gas and drive away? Both premium and economy gas options get your car moving, although premium blends cost more and claim to be better for your engine. The same analogy can be made between the two types of food that fuel your body. You have different ways to "gas up" your body's engine—you either run on economy gas (glucose) or make premium gas (ketones). There! That makes sense, right?

What's wrong with the cheap gas—glucose? Everybody loves glucose! Glucose is a by-product of eating carbohydrates. Glucose is simply blood sugar; in fact, the Greek word for sweet is *glykys*. Whether you eat brown rice or a cookie (despite one tasting healthier than the other), both are quickly converted by the body into glucose. So not fair!

Glucose fuels your engine, true, but for many of us who are overweight, our engines process glucose differently (and perhaps inefficiently). When we eat foods that are rich in carbohydrates, our body responds by converting carbs into a cheap, quick glucose supply. Led by its overzealous leader, the hormone *insulin,* glucose swims around in our blood fueling various body systems. That sounds good, right? But like all good things, accepting glucose as a fuel source must be done in moderation. That's where our problems start. People like you and me *do not eat carbs in moderation.* Why is that?

Unlike the gas pump that shuts off when the tank is full, the body just keeps accepting more fuel. When we overload on carbohydrates, too often the body overproduces glucose and insulin, causing a backup. Now the body is smart and doesn't want to waste this surplus energy. It holds on to this excess for a rainy day, storing the converted glucose to a longer-lasting energy source: FAT. This efficient hoarding strategy is probably left over from our Neanderthal days, when meals were sporadic.

Is this biological process our fault? No! The overproduction of glucose and insulin is not caused from personal weakness around food or a lack of willpower. This is where I call *bullshit*. I'm so tired of the judgment and shame society places on those of us who struggle with our weight.

Metabolically, there is more at play here than just my own inability to put down the chips.

I would like to propose a novel idea here. What if there is something wrong with insulin, the hormone I mentioned earlier, in the obese? I'm going to go off on a tangent, but bear with me. There is a growing movement among researchers looking at insulin sensitivity and its role in losing weight. People who are more "sensitive" to their insulin are able to digest a higher level of carbohydrates (but not store excess glucose as fat). These are the thin people *we all hate,* who can eat anything and never gain weight. I am not one of those people, and I suspect neither are you.

Conversely, when you have a "weak" response to insulin (like me), you are called "insulin resistant." Even though my body is trying to tell me that I am full, *I can't hear the voice.* I just keep eating. I have no "off switch." Intellectually, I know that overeating is not good for me, but my body physically doesn't agree with me. I rarely feel full. For example, I can eat an entire extra-large tub of popcorn at the movies (*and maybe the free refill, too, if I'm being 100 percent honest!*). Why is my brain like this? Why can't I just stop eating, like other people do?

I promised I wouldn't get "all scientifical" *(yup, I made that one up!),* so I'm going to wrap this up. At this time, there is no cure for being insulin resistant. It tends to worsen with age and is thought to be related to additional uncontrollable factors like genetics, a family history of diabetes, or even your ethnicity. This is *SO NOT FAIR*, and I'd like to be the first to acknowledge this point. We are not "normal," like those people who can *share* a small popcorn. (*That's just weird.*) To all the naturally thin people frowning at me in line at the concession stand when I order an extra-large tub of popcorn, let me tell you this:

**No amount of willpower or fat shaming will
change my inner metabolism.**

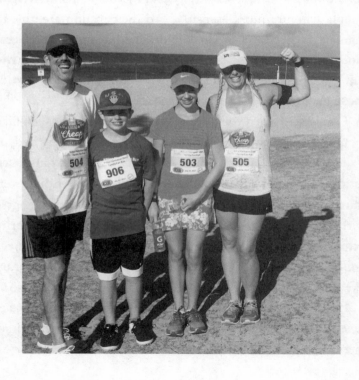

All this being said, I have found that DIRTY, LAZY, KETO helped me beat the odds and overcome these almost *insurmountable challenges,* and with long-lasting results. Ketosis—no matter how you achieve this fat-burning state— might just be the cure to obesity.

Are you convinced? Let's get started then. How about we take a look at the keto jargon that will be thrown around later? This is like a secret handshake that will help you fit in to your new keto tribe.

Glossary

As a courtesy, I've included an alphabetized glossary of commonly used words and phrases. Keep in mind that my definition of these keto-related terms might be different from what you have heard before.

Bi-Strict Keto dieters lurk in the middle ground between strict and dirty. Isn't this fun? Bi-strict keto dieters go back and forth, becoming stricter (if needed) to break a weight-loss stall, or just to "mix it up." They might "eat clean" most of the time, but allow for little treats like a Diet Coke or low-carb ice cream once in a while. While their belief system is different from mine, I admire how bi-strict keto dieters are doing what works for them. I recognize my way isn't the only way; flexibility and style are important. Keto on, I say to these folks! Let's hang out.

DIRTY, LAZY, KETO is not just a diet, it's a lifestyle. As a modern hybrid, it reaps the benefits of losing weight, but without limitations of food choices or the obligation of counting every macro. We are open to the idea of artificial sweeteners (Diet Coke or Splenda, for example) and include packaged foods (protein bars, low-carb tortillas) in our meals. Dirty and lazy keto followers focus on the big picture of daily net carbs consumption. I am the superhero of this category! I even coined the term. Somebody make me a T-shirt!

Dirty Keto is eating whatever foods you choose within your macro goals or limits (which are different for everyone). Dirty keto has a reputation (which may or may not be true) of including junk food in its diet (no judgment!). For example, if you want to eat a hot dog, then have at it. This is your body, and only you can decide what to eat or drink. Dirty keto means you can play dirty and don't have to follow specific rules about your eating (other than the "big picture" of counting macros). Artificial sweeteners and low-carb substitutes are fair game. Dirty keto followers don't limit their food or beverage choices and might even be spotted drinking a Diet Coke (oh, the horror!).

Dirty Strict Keto followers are not as regimented with their ingredient choices. They still identify as strict because they prefer to count all of their macros (fat, protein, carbs) and maybe even calories. Dirty Strict is flexible and open-minded. They aren't afraid of artificial sweeteners, grain-based fillers, chemical additives, or sugar substitutes.

Keto is simply a shortened word for "ketogenic." It sounds a bit sexier and less medical, so let's go with that.

Ketogenic Diet is a diet of foods that are low in carbohydrates, moderate in protein, and higher in fat, with the goal of one's body going into ketosis.

Keto Police, are my archnemeses. Where I am inclusive, they are judgmental. Like members of a cult, the Keto Police passionately cling to their "right" version of keto and shame anyone who disagrees. They believe their way is the only way and will publicly flog defectors or those that stray. Though they don't wear a uniform, you can easily spot a member of the Keto Police for their social media posts that frequently ridicule others, arguing, "but THAT'S NOT KETO!" Keto Police believe their sanctity makes them superior; they constantly feel the need to educate and "correct" dissenting keto methods.

Keto Purists are the most extreme of all keto followers: They completely avoid artificial or chemically processed foods and may demand absolute organic, natural whole-food ingredients. These good soldiers take great pride in following "the rules." Keto purists pay meticulous close attention to every detail. They count carbs from just a splash of soy sauce or even a sugar-free cough drop. Keto purists document calories in addition to ongoing calculations of macro goals and limits. Needless to say, these folks don't like me very much!

Lazy Keto followers only count their net carbs intake—not fat grams or protein intake. Lazy keto does NOT mean unwilling to work hard for weight loss. This term refers to just one style of counting a single macro in keto—the net carb—not a relaxed lifestyle or lack of energy. Not tracking doesn't mean overconsumption, though! Common sense is always used.

Strict Keto adheres to a rigid and closely monitored diet constructed of intentional fat, calorie, protein, and carbohydrate goals. There are multiple factions within strict keto: Keto Purists, Dirty-Strict Keto, Bi-Strict Keto, and the most intimidating of all . . . the Keto Police!

If you are still not sure what keto camp you fall into, try taking the free, short quiz I created on my website at https://dirtylazyketo.com/quiz/.

Related Terms

A1C is a simple, non-fasting, virtually painless medical test used to evaluate blood glucose levels over the past 2–3 months, which helps physicians determine if a patient has (or is heading toward) diabetes.

"Counting Macros" is how many keto dieters track their intake of macronutrients (proteins, fats, and carbohydrates); instead of counting calories, you'll hear the phrase "counting macros" often in keto-land. Dieters might have a goal or a limit for each category, or a specific ratio to achieve each day with their eating choices. Apps and food calculators can be used to track daily food choices if it helps for accuracy and motivation. Everyone goes about this in a slightly different way. Note that the only macro I ever counted were net carbohydrates. I kept a mental tally in my head throughout the day.

Calories are units of heat that food provides to the body. There are no "good" or "bad" calories. You've got to let this one go, people! A calorie is just an innocent unit of measurement, like a cup or a gallon. Our bodies REQUIRE calories to survive. With DIRTY, LAZY, KETO, calories are not the focus (instead, net carbs). The 1980s are over, my friends, and only counting calories of low-fat foods is just as passé as leg warmers.

Carbohydrates, or "Carbs" (for short), are sugars, starches, and fibers found in fruits, grains, vegetables, and milk products. Foods high in carbs include bread, pasta, beans, potatoes, rice, grains, and cereals. In general, packaged or processed foods from your pantry are likely high in carb content. Carbs contain four calories per gram. To further break down this macro group, I reclassified carbs into two unique sub-categories: Fast-burning carbs and Slow-burning carbs.

Fast-burning carbs are simple sugars that quickly release glucose into the bloodstream. These include processed carbohydrates like breads, cereals, sugars, high-sugar fruits, and some starchy vegetables. Common examples are candy, soda, pasta, potatoes, popcorn, tortillas, corn, and bananas. This is the category of foods that has caused me (and I suspect you, too) so much trouble!

Slow-burning carbs have a high-fiber content and lower glycemic index. They are less likely to cause a spike in blood sugar. Slow-burning carbs are more desirable (in my opinion), as they keep you feeling fuller for longer. They offer your body better overall health benefits when compared to fast-burning carbs. Examples of foods that have slow-burning carbs are non-starchy, high-fiber vegetables like celery or broccoli. Slow-burning carbs are your weight-loss best friends! They are more conducive to your overall well-being than simple, fast-burning carbs because they help maintain a steady blood sugar state and don't cause a backlash of sugar cravings.

Chaffle is a modern portmanteau meaning "cheese waffle." This glorious, addictive bread substitute is made in just a few minutes using a handful of ingredients and cooked inside a waffle iron.

Fat Bombs are low-carb, artificially sweetened, high-fat desserts.

Fats are the densest form of energy, providing nine calories per gram. The most obvious example of fat is oil (olive, coconut, sesame, canola, vegetable oil, etc.). Less clear examples of fats are dairy foods, nuts, avocados, and oily fish. Some fats have a better reputation than others. (Think about how the media portrays eggs, mayonnaise, alfredo sauce, or chicken skin.) No matter what the quality of the source, fat is fat is fat.

Fiber is not digested by the body and is removed as waste. There are two types of fiber, soluble and insoluble.

Insoluble Fiber does NOT absorb water. Insoluble fiber moves through the intestine mostly intact, adding bulk to the stool.

Keto Flu is an avoidable set of symptoms (headache, lethargy, leg cramps) associated with dehydration, often experienced at the onset of the keto diet. Because the metabolic process of ketosis requires more water, increased hydration is required by the body.

Ketone Urine–Testing Strips are just what you might expect. They are little strips of paper that, when dipped in your urine, will identify if your body has reached ketosis, or weight-loss mode. I have never used a ketone urine-testing strip in my life, but I wanted to let you know about their availability. I suspect just getting on the scale might be cheaper than buying these (and less messy—just sayin').

Ketones are acids. Ketones are present when fat is breaking down. Ketones are often found in the blood and urine during weight loss.

Ketosis occurs when the body burns ketones from the liver as the main energy source (as opposed to using glucose as the energy source, derived from carbs). Ketosis is often an indicator (but not a requirement) of weight loss.

LCHF Diet consists of eating low-carbohydrate, high-fat foods (acronym) without the goal of ketosis. You may be totally shocked to learn that some slender folks eat LCHF for reasons other than weight loss. Benefits of eating LCHF might include a reduction of inflammation, decreased joint pain, increased energy, or the ability to maintain weight loss.

Macronutrients, or "**Macros,**" come in three forms: carbohydrates, protein, and fat. All macronutrients are obtained through foods in the diet, as the body cannot produce them. Macronutrients are necessary for fuel. There are no "good" macros or "bad" macros (though one of them is definitely my favorite—ahhh, carboliciousness). Each macro fulfills vital roles with nutrition and your health. All macros contain calories, but at different densities.

Net Carbs are the unit of measurement tracked in DIRTY, LAZY, KETO. When looking at a nutrition label, net carbs are calculated by subtracting all fiber grams and sugar alcohol grams (more on sugar alcohols later!) from the listed amount of carbohydrates. Total carbs, minus fiber, minus sugar alcohol equals net carbs. Net carbs are the carbs left over in this mathematical equation. (Sugar, as a side note, is NOT subtracted; sorry!)

Protein has four calories per gram. Proteins take longer to digest because they are long-chain amino acids. Protein is largely found in meats, dairy foods, eggs, legumes, nuts, and seafood.

Soluble Fiber absorbs water. When you eat foods high in soluble fiber it turns to mush inside your body. Soluble fiber absorbs water quickly and helps to soften your stool while adding bulk.

Sugar Alcohols are reduced-calorie sweeteners, but they do not contain alcohol. They are commonly used in sugar-free candy and low-carb desserts.

Common Keto Abbreviations

AS—Artificial Sweetener
BMI—Body Mass Index
BPC—Bulletproof Coffee
CDC—Center for Disease Control
CW—Current Weight
DLK—DIRTY, LAZY, KETO
FDA—U.S. Federal Drug Administration
GW—Goal Weight
HWC—Heavy Whipping Cream
IF—Intermittent Fasting
IIFIYM—If It Fits in Your Macros
LC—Low-Carb
MCT—Medium-Chain Triglyceride, as in MCT Oil
NSV—Non-Scale Victory
OMAD—One Meal a Day
PCOS—Polycystic Ovarian Syndrome
RDA—Recommended Daily Allowance
SA—Sugar Alcohol
SAD—Standard American Diet
SF—Sugar-Free
SV—Scale Victory
SW—Starting Weight
USDA—United States Department of Agriculture

WOE—Way of Eating
WOL—Way of Living

I just threw a lot of vocabulary at you, so take a breath and maybe even a break. Some of this might be new information for you to think about. I'm guessing you might even have strong opinions about what you have just read. *Good . . . great!* That's what makes this plan so wonderful. You can tweak it to your heart's content. Personalize the hell out of it. Make it work for YOU.

**I only want to share with you WHAT WORKED FOR ME.
You can follow in my size 9 footsteps or blaze
your own trail beside me.**

My only ask is that we stick together and support one another. Let's not judge each other for our personal tastes, budgets, or lifestyles.

DIRTY, LAZY, KETO works best for me when I eat between 20 and 50 grams of net carbs per day. This is a big range, people! Some days (or weeks) I eat toward the lower end of the net carbs range (20 grams), and some days, at the higher end (50 grams). Why is that? Was there some calculated nutritional plan at work? NOPE! While I was losing 140 pounds, I did not have a strict plan. Real life was happening while I was trying to lose weight, and I needed some breathing room to account for roadblocks, challenges, and the dips in my motivation. Ultimately, by giving myself some wiggle room, I created a flexible environment where I could still be successful. Was I in ketosis every single second? *Probably not.* But in the big picture, which mattered most to me, I lost weight. It was *freaking* magical!

Everyone asks me, "HOW LONG DID IT TAKE?" What they are secretly wishing for here is for a magic wand to melt away their fat instantaneously. I understand.

While I may have said all of this in the beginning, it doesn't hurt to remind you again, my dear reader, THAT THIS REALLY WORKS. I lost around 10 pounds a month for about a year and a half. I lost 140 pounds total. Isn't that INSANE? I literally lost about half of my entire body. *That's a little freaky, even.*

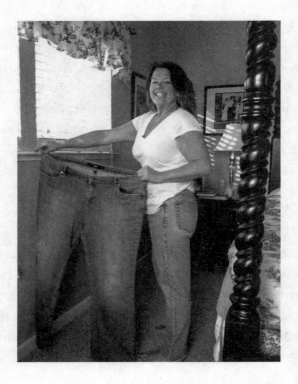

The weirdest part (I don't want to jinx myself here) was that *it wasn't that hard*. Please don't slam the book shut at this point and run from the room yelling, "This girl is CRAAAAAAAZY!" I'm being serious. Once I figured out what I was doing (like how to read a nutrition label), the whole thing just flowed for me. Yes, there were obstacles along the way, but looking at the big picture, I quickly realized that this was a way I could really eat, *like forever,* and be happy! I'm betting you can do this, too, with great success.

Let's get specific now. For starters, I didn't write anything down. I didn't track anything with an app or even a pencil. In hindsight I realize I might have tempted fate with that strategy! I think I might have PTSD from my Weight Watchers days where I calculated and documented points in an official booklet. That made me crazy, I'll tell you. I would lie and cheat, borrow and steal (from myself, mind you) with that tracker, and this time, I didn't want a repeat performance. That was me, though, and not you. I recommend that you follow whatever method will keep you, in all your honest glory, accountable. If you need to write down every morsel of what you're eating to be successful, then you should definitely do it!

Now what about counting the other "macros" besides carbs? I'll be honest here. Other than focusing on eating within a range 20–50 grams of net carbs a day, I didn't count anything else, not a calorie nor a fat gram. (That's lazy keto, folks.) I didn't have a "goal" or a "minimum" to achieve each day for fats or proteins. Instead, I added fat and protein to every meal. We can get into that more, later. For now, though, I want to provide a broad picture of *what* I did and *why* I think it was successful.

Is there a reason why I didn't count fat or protein grams? Or impose goals or limits? Well, for me, all that counting and tracking just sounded exhausting and intimidating. I was already having a monumental lifestyle adjustment by breaking up with the love of my life, carbohydrates. Piling on more rules or required steps sounded overwhelming and could become that one excuse for me to give up. Besides, what I was doing was already working: I was losing weight!

Prior to eating DIRTY, LAZY, KETO, my daily carb intake was *ridiculously* high. Pasta, bread, cereal, rice: The staples of my frugal family meals were overwhelmed with carbs. Ironically, I actually considered myself a healthy eater. I didn't eat a lot of junk food or desserts. I only drank Diet Coke and often snacked on baby carrots or bags of "whole wheat" Crunchy Corn Bran, for cryin' out loud.

I was ignorant about how carbs affected my mood and energy level. Unbeknownst to me, every time I ate a carb-rich food, my body went into overdrive, producing glucose and a quick spike in my blood sugar. In my brain, dopamine (the "feel good" hormone and neurotransmitter) was released. The immediate physical response from eating carbs was (*and still is!*) pure, unadulterated pleasure. This positive physical reaction is why I couldn't stop!

This pleasurable response, however, was short-lived. Massive amounts of insulin were secreted to counteract the high level of sugar coursing through my blood, leading my body to store glucose as fat. *Well, that's not fair!* Then, to make matters even more complicated, lowered blood sugar levels led to moodiness and a desire to eat again. These reactions caused the entire cycle to repeat itself, ALL DAY LONG, resulting in excessive calorie intake. *No wonder I weighed so much.*

Simply reducing my net carbs intake to a range of 20–50 grams per day had an immediate effect on my weight and overall energy levels. Instead of eating meals and snacks mainly of carbs all day, I ate protein, *slow-burning carbs,* and healthy fats. This new combination caused many changes, all for the better. *I felt energetic, consistently full, and much happier!*

One thing that shocked the hell out of me was the effects of eating protein. I suspected eating fats wouldn't be a problem. (Who doesn't like cheese?) But I was surprised to discover how eating more proteins at every meal made such a difference. I didn't find myself overeating protein like I did with simple carbs. If I ate protein at a meal or for a snack, I would actually feel fuller for longer. By choosing slow-burning carbs, my body surprisingly experienced more sustained energy. I wouldn't feel sleepy after eating a meal. My frequent headaches suddenly stopped. The afternoon exhaustion, the moodiness—gone.

Whoa . . . Shit just got real (excuse my language).

The dramatic improvement in my overall health—not just my weight loss—is what compels me to share my story!

If I can help even one person climb out of the carbohydrate-laden hole that they have dug themselves into, stopping the horrible cycle of feeling like crap all the time, then this will all have been worth it. *(Sorry, starting to well up a bit here.)*

DIRTY, LAZY, KETO is a simple solution to the "food part" of the weight-loss riddle. It's sustainable. It's flexible. There are no magic shakes, required pills, or strict rules to abide by. The low-carb, moderate-protein, higher fat foods give you consistent energy, reduce inflammation, and help the body run more efficiently. It's a fairy-tale food ending we've all been looking for.

But is losing weight THAT simple? If cutting carbs were the cure to obesity, we'd all just stop eating bread and candy, and life would be perfect—*right*?

Implementing a new way of eating definitely brings about new challenges, and none have to do with food! Have you ever lost ten pounds but caved when faced with a pushy relative offering a piece of cake, "because you deserve it"? Have you ever lost your ability to "rebound" after a self-identified "cheat meal"? These weight-loss obstacles (and the hundreds of others!) will be explored in this essential support guide. *DIRTY, LAZY, KETO* is not just about food—*it's a complete lifestyle.*

Learn from my mistakes. Changing eating habits isn't effective if behaviors and your state of mind don't evolve at the same time. Let me help inspire and support you as you begin your own weight-loss journey. Get your camera out now to take a mirror selfie, because soon you will be amazed at your own before-and-after weight-loss photos.

Not to be cheesy or anything, but I'm really excited to partner with you right now. DIRTY, LAZY, KETO is life-changing and transformative. Scoot over, friend. You're going to need a buddy, because *this is going to be a wild ride!*

Count the Carbs That Matter

I once received an email from a desperate dieter who was "totally freaked out" over the number of calories she was eating. She went on and on with detailed graphs, charts, and lists of foods she ate that day. The total number of calories she consumed was written at the bottom of the email, followed by a series of exclamation points—!!!!! She was panicking.

I understand how scary it is to make a big change like this. The whole concept of eating fat seemed unnatural to me, too! I was brought up hearing the message that only a "low-fat" calorie-restrictive diet would lead to weight loss. The DIRTY, LAZY, KETO way of eating was the exact *opposite* of what I had been taught as a child. Additionally, I never felt hungry. That seemed suspicious! I identified with the uncertainty she felt. How could this work? I encouraged her to take a leap of faith—and trust the process. DIRTY, LAZY, KETO works!

I didn't count calories or use fancy apps to make unnecessary graphs. I learned to read food labels and focused on eating high-fiber, low-carbohydrate foods with healthy fats and protein at every meal. **I ate actual food.** I didn't try and "game the system" with cheat days, chowing down on keto junk food, or drinking exogenous ketones* (waste of money). While

---

* Marketed as a "quick fix," exogenous ketones are supplements dieters take with hopes of rushing their body into a state of ketosis. Aggressive online multilevel marketers often

I love Moon Cheese, Quest Chips, and Atkins Bars, I know those convenience foods ultimately leave me unsatisfied, broke, and—if we are being transparent here—*constipated*. I realize it's your choice to eat these kinds of foods. You might fight back on this one, for sure! But if your weight loss starts to stall out, come back to this part of the book for a second read. Maybe then you'll be more motivated to cut back on keto goodies.

I used fats to make healthy food taste better. I kept a mental tally of my total net carbs for the day. I chose a re-alistic range of net carbs, which for me was between 20 and 50 grams of net carbs per day. This range made sense for my own body/activity level. Ultimately, I cut my body weight in half. This works!

Reading a food label with DIRTY, LAZY, KETO rules might be different from what you've been taught. Before I send you out into the real world of eating, let's test your knowledge. In my version of keto-land, net carbs are counted by starting with total carbs and then subtracting any grams of fiber and/or sugar alcohols.* Multiply the remaining num-ber by the serving size (*the most important part!*) that you eat. The end result is your net carbs. Net carbs are what you "count" in your daily allotment.

"Allowing" sugar alcohols is unique to DIRTY, LAZY, KETO. Many strict keto or "true keto" supporters (their words, *not mine!*) find sugar alcohols distasteful or down-

---

prey on the vulnerabilities of desperate dieters by promoting unnecessary exogenous ketone supplements.

* Fiber and sugar alcohols are not digested the same way as other carbohydrates are; they move very quickly through your digestive system. This explains why they have less of an impact on your blood sugar levels.

right dangerous. I would like to tip my hat in acknowledgment to these criticisms. I'd like to address the naysayers, so let me climb onto my soapbox for a moment.

The FDA has deemed sugar alcohols and sugar substitutes as GRAS (generally recognized as safe). Therefore, they are "certifiably" approved for you to use. I understand that this U.S. stamp of approval doesn't mean sugar alcohols are healthy or nutritious, just that they are "safe" to eat. Whether or not you trust the government is up to you, but that being said, I am willing to take my chances by eating them. Without these "sugar crutches," I can 100 percent guarantee I would've fallen back into my old habits of eating excessive amounts of harmful sweets. For me, eating sugar leads to gaining weight—*excessive weight gain*! Obesity comes with its own set of detrimental health issues, like type 2 diabetes, so I am going to pick between the two evils. I'd rather eat Splenda than give myself insulin shots. *My body, my choice.*

Sugar alcohols are not perfect by any means. Some cause unanticipated reactions. As long as sugar alcohols or sugar substitutes don't cause you any dietary distress (flatulence, diarrhea, etc.), then I support your common-sense approach to using them as a tool to help you lose weight. Additionally, if you find these ingredients cause an unexpected increase in your hunger or sugar cravings, then obviously discontinue their use (or limit your exposure).

I wish I could eat real sugars (in any of their forms) in safe amounts, I really do. Sadly, even natural sugars (agave, honey, etc.) cause me the same problem. Sugar causes me to completely lose control. I am not able to stop myself from overeating anything that is sweet. Even at my current healthier weight, I sometimes crave sugary treats.

I am still an emotional eater, a stress eater, and even a celebratory eater, and by choosing to incorporate some sugar alcohols and sugar substitutes when needed, I am still able to maintain my weight loss.

Like many of us who struggle with obesity and carb addiction, I am probably insulin resistant. Note that many scientists don't acknowledge insulin resistance is a "thang"; rather, many medical professionals continue to hold on to the erroneous belief that obesity stems from a lack of willpower. To make sure I'm heard on this point, I am now about to shout very loudly (*cover your ears*): THEY COULD NOT BE MORE WRONG!

Effects of Insulin Resistance

I will lay out the effects of insulin resistance for you quite simply:

If you are new to the keto lifestyle, you might be wondering how I could eat low-carb, high-fat foods (which are potentially higher in calories) and still lose weight. I wondered about this, too, when I started. The foods enjoyed on DIRTY, LAZY, KETO rebel against every weight-loss rule you've

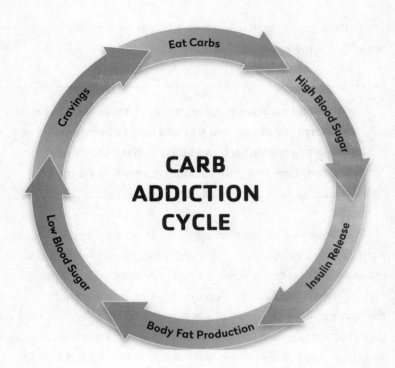

CARB ADDICTION CYCLE

Eat Carbs → High Blood Sugar → Insulin Release → Body Fat Production → Low Blood Sugar → Cravings

probably been taught! Enjoying these "naughty" foods feels scandalous, right?

Eating fat to lose weight is a secret of the DIRTY, LAZY, KETO lifestyle. Scientists are the first to admit that they don't understand how metabolism actually works. There is still much to be learned in the medical community about nutrition and weight loss. To put DIRTY, LAZY, KETO in perspective, however, let's take a look at the current mainstream nutritional standards.

U.S. *Dietary Guidelines for Americans* (published jointly by the Health and Human Services and Department of

Agriculture) recommends that carbs make up 45–65 percent of total calories consumed.* That translates to around 300 CARBS PER DAY! The standard American diet (or SAD, how ironic) reflects the belief that eating whole grains is the foundation of healthy eating: breads, pasta, potatoes, and cereal. I'm sure these "experts" have good intentions when recommending we eat six to eight servings per day of whole-grain starches, but it seems that there is a disconnect. Despite following "the guidelines," nearly 40 percent of adult Americans and 18.5 percent of all children are obese!† Type 2 diabetes, a direct complication of obesity, has reached epidemic levels. Is there a connection? *I say yes.*

Even though I hold many answers, I don't think anyone in government is listening (*shocking, I know!*). I logged my incredible weight-loss results with the National Weight Control Registry. (Who knew this was a thing?) I assumed that my phone would ring off the hook from researchers wanting clues on how to solve the weight-loss riddle. That never happened. No one has called. *(Cue sound effect of tap, tap, tap of fingers on desk.)*

Like Cindy Lou Who from Whoville,‡ I'm shouting as loud as I can. I've started my own grass-roots campaign to help others fight obesity, one net carb at a time. To start, I'll teach you how to accurately read a nutrition label.

---

* https://health.gov/dietaryguidelines/2015/resources/2015-2020_Dietary_Guidelines.pdf.
† www.cdc.gov/obesity/index.html.
‡ Cindy Lou Who from Whoville is a character from *How the Grinch Stole Christmas!* by Dr. Seuss.

How to Read a Nutrition Label on
DIRTY, LAZY, KETO

Nutrition Facts

Serving Size 1/2 cup (64g)
Serving Per Container 4

Amount Per Serving

Calories 80	Calories from Fat 25

% Daily Value*

Total Fat 2.5g	4%
Saturated Fat 1.5g	8%
Trans Fat 0g	
Cholesterol 45mg	15%
Sodium 110mg	5%
Total Carbohydrate 13g	4%
Dietary Fiber 2g	
Sugars 6g	
Sugar Alcohol 5g	
Protein 5g	

Vitamin A 2%	Vitamin C 0%
Calcium 10%	Iron 2%

* Percent Daily Values are based on a 2,000-calorie diet

*Sugar Alcohols affect everyone differently. Enjoy with caution.

❶ Notice the serving size

❷ Find the Total Carbohydrate number **13**

❸ Subtract the amount of Dietary fiber **−2**

❹ Subtract the amount of Sugar Alcohol *(if applicable) **−5**

The result is the **NET CARBS** per serving. For more help visit **www.DIRTYLAZYKETO.com** ⑥

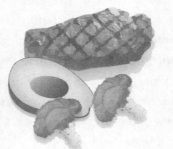

Celery vs. Coffee Creamer:
Are All Carbs Created Equal?

Some carbs keep you feeling fuller, for longer, than others. For example, celery and coffee creamer both have the same amount of carbs, which is about 1 gram of carbs per serving. Does that seem fair? Does this comparison even make sense? It would seem to an outsider (or my low-fat-dieting grandmother) that one of these foods is drastically healthier than the other. I beg to differ.

Celery, an example of a healthy, slow-burning carb, is leisurely metabolized. The fiber keeps you feeling full for longer. Cruciferous vegetables (cauliflower, broccoli, and cabbage, to name a few) are the poster children for slow-burning carbs and will play a starring role throughout this book. At every turn possible, I aim to increase the amount of healthy, slow-burning carbs in my snacks and meals. *Learn to love these weight-loss beauties, and watch excess weight fall off.*

Is celery the clear winner over creamer? Not so fast. Surprisingly, fats play a pivotal role in the DIRTY, LAZY, KETO lifestyle. Fats help keep you satiated. They make you feel scandalous—*like you aren't on a diet.* Fat tastes good! Who eats cheese or sour cream and still loses weight? I DO! How weird is that?

Enjoying fats is encouraged on DIRTY LAZY, KETO, but not to excess; after all, you are trying to burn the fat from your booty, not the venti Starbucks drink that you just downed, right? Don't go overboard on the fats, whether it be in a fat bomb or your bulletproof coffee. Go ahead and cancel that order for the Starbucks Pink Drink, as eating fat only for fat's sake is not recommended here.

How should you eat your fat, then, if not in a fat bomb? Lean in, my friend, because what I'm about to tell you is truly one of the secrets of adulthood, if not the key to sustainable weight loss. The French have known this for years, but us Americans? We have struggled in this area. **The path to sustainable weight loss on DIRTY, LAZY, KETO is to enjoy fat** (*wait for it, wait for it . . .*) **with VEGETABLES!** Butter and

Brussels sprouts, bacon and cheese–topped cauliflower, green beans with sliced almonds—the combinations of these satisfying pairs are endless and all support sustainable weight loss.

Are you surprised or repelled by hearing this secret? I know, I know, this is DIRTY, LAZY, KETO, and technically, you can eat whatever you want, but I urge you to consider my personal secret sauce for making weight loss last. Were you expecting some other answer? **If you plan on keeping your weight off and turning your life around, the sooner you get over any *vegetable anxiety* the better.**

Vegetables are seriously the magic ingredient for making your weight-loss dreams come true. *Romance them* and *get to know* your vegetables. Dress them up in butter, ghee, oil, cheese, sour cream, ANYTHING to help you eat lots of vegetables. Eat vegetables as if your life depends on it (*because maybe it does!*). They are full of fiber and life-sustaining vitamins and minerals that prevent illness and keep you healthy. They also make you feel full and help melt away excess body fat. Vegetables are the prizewinning, slow-burning carbs that will wake up your sluggish metabolism.

While plants are the stars of DIRTY, LAZY, KETO, protein and fats play Oscar-winning supporting roles. Personally, I eat some protein and fat with every meal, but without a specific goal or limit in mind. Seriously—no measuring or counting, I just add some to my meals.

Will the range of 20–50 grams of net carbs work the same for everyone? *Absolutely not!* We come from varying starting weights and different activity levels, so there will be *no magic number* that universally applies to everyone. In fact, when you hear someone purporting otherwise, an alarm bell should go off. Our bodies are unique. You might even find that you can eat more than 20–50 grams of net carbs when you first start DIRTY, LAZY, KETO, and still lose weight! Crazy, right?

Before I started following a DIRTY, LAZY, KETO diet, I likely consumed 700, 800, maybe even 1,000 carbs every day! Before you start judging me (or denying that's possible), take a look at the net carb count of commonly eaten foods. (These numbers are per serving; *you know how small those usually are!*) I understand these might not be foods that you are currently eating, but they certainly were part of my regular diet *back in the day*. I have to laugh at myself, because I actually thought *some* of my choices (especially the breakfast foods) were "healthy" (NOT!). Wow, what a wake-up call!

As a courtesy, throughout the book I try to provide you with the most accurate nutrition information possible. Finding accurate nutrition information often proved challenging due to the number of discrepancies between reference sites. *So frustrating!* Before coming up with final numbers to include here, I compared nutrition information from a variety of sources: Carb Manager App,* USDA,† actual food labels at local grocery stores, product websites, and lastly—*common sense*! If something doesn't seem right—trust your instincts and check another source. I encourage you to independently research the nutrition of what you eat. It's been my experience that ingredients and serving sizes vary widely across brands.

---

* https://www.carbmanager.com/
† https://www.usda.gov/

1,000 Carbs a Day? The Traditional American Diet Is Making Us Fat

High-Carb Foods I Used to Eat

High-Carb Breakfast Items

Bagel, 53 g net carbs per medium serving (3½" to 4" in diameter)

Biscuit, 16 g net carbs per medium serving (2½" in diameter)

Blueberry muffin, 48 g net carbs per medium serving (2¾" to 3" in diameter)

Bran muffin, 44 g net carbs per medium serving (2¾" to 3" in diameter)

Canned pineapple in juice (not drained), 18 g net carbs per 1 cup serving

Cinnamon roll (with raisins, commercially prepared), 40 g net carbs per single large serving

Cornflakes, 23 g net carbs per 1 cup serving

Cream of Wheat (instant), 192 g net carbs per 1 (1 oz.) packet serving

Crepe (fruit-filled), 19 g net carbs per 78 g serving

Croissant, 26 g net carbs per medium serving (4½" in diameter)

Donut (plain), 25 g net carbs per medium serving (3¼" in diameter)

English muffin, 23 g net carbs per whole serving (3½" in diameter)

French toast, 14 g net carbs per medium slice, using white bread

Grits, 36 g net carbs per 1 cup serving

Hash browns, 24 g net carbs per ½ cup serving

Homestyle potatoes (O'Brien-style), 20 g net carbs per ½ cup serving

Jelly, jam, and preserves, 13 g net carbs per 1 tablespoon serving

Maple syrup, 53 g net carbs per ¼ cup serving

Nutella, 21 g net carbs per 2 tablespoon serving

Oatmeal (regular cooked), 24 g net carbs per 1 cup serving

Orange juice, 25 g net carbs per 8 fl. oz. serving

Pancake syrup, 55 g net carbs per ¼ cup serving

Pancakes, 39 g net carbs per serving of 3 pancakes 4" in diameter

Pastry (fruit-filled Danish), 51 g net carbs per medium serving (4¼" in diameter)

Pop-Tarts, 37 g net carbs per 1 pastry serving (52 gram)

Raisin bran cereal, 40 g net carbs per 1 cup serving

Strawberry yogurt (nonfat), 28 g net carbs per 1 cup serving

Toast (white or wheat), 13 g net carbs per 1 medium slice serving

Waffles, 30 g net carbs per 1 medium serving (7" in diameter)

High-Carb Snacks

Banana, 24 g net carbs per 1 serving of a whole, medium-sized fruit

Candy Corn, 46 g net carbs per 24 pieces serving

Cheez-It crackers, 28 g net carbs per serving of 1 cup

Cherries (fresh), 18 g net carbs per serving of 1 cup

Dates, 25 g net carbs per serving of ¼ cup

Doritos, 14 g net carbs per 1 oz. serving

Dried cranberries, 31 g net carbs per ¼ cup

Goldfish crackers, 19 g net carbs per 55 piece serving

Granola bar, 26 g net carbs per 2 (.75 oz.) bar serving

Grapes, 26 g net carbs per 1 cup serving

Hershey's Kisses (milk chocolate), 18 g net carbs per 7 piece serving

Instant noodles, 71 g net carbs per 1 cup serving

Oatmeal raisin cookie, 21 g net carbs per 2 cookies (2⅕″ in diameter) serving

Party Mix (cereal), 19 g net carbs per ½ cup serving

Peanut butter cookie, 22 g net carbs per 2 cookies (3″ in diameter) serving

Pineapple (fresh), 19 g net carbs per 1 cup serving

Popcorn, 43 g net carbs per 1 (2.75 oz.) microwaved popped bag serving

Potato chips, 14 g net carbs per 1 oz. serving

Pretzels, 22 g net carbs per 1 oz. serving

Prunes (dried), 19 g net carbs per ¼ cup serving

Rice cakes, 21 g net carbs per 3 regular cakes (4″ in diameter) serving

Rice Krispies Treats, 25 g net carbs per 1 square serving (4″ × 4″)

Ritz Crackers (original), 17 g net carbs per 9 cracker serving

Saltine crackers (original), 21 g net carbs per 10 cracker serving

Snickers bar, 34 g net carbs per 1 (2 oz.) bar serving

Tortilla chips, 17 g net carbs per 1 oz. serving

Triscuit crackers (original), 17 g net carbs per 6 cracker serving

Wheat Thins (original), 18 g net carbs per 15 cracker serving

High-Carb Meal Items

Baked potato, 26 g net carbs per medium-sized serving (2¼″ to 3″ in diameter)

Barbecue sauce, 14 g net carbs per 2 tablespoon serving

Bean-and-cheese burrito, 33 g net carbs per 1 (6″ × 8″ in diameter) folded tortilla for a 6.3 oz. serving

Black beans, 13 g net carbs per ½ cup serving

Bread (wheat), 26 g net carbs per 2 medium slice serving

Bread (white), 26 g net carbs per 2 medium slice serving

Breadstick, 15 g net carbs per 1 medium (6¾" long) serving

Brown rice, 48 g net carbs per 1 cup serving

Cheese lasagna, 45 g net carbs per 1 cup serving

Corn dog (mini), 25 g net carbs per 5 servings.

Corn on the cob, 19 g net carbs per 1 medium ear (6¾" to 7½" long) serving

Creamed canned corn, 22 g net carbs per ½ cup serving

Dinner roll, 22 g net carbs per 1 medium roll (2½" in diameter) serving

Enchilada (cheese, no beans or meat), 14 g net carbs per 1 (6" in diameter) tortilla rolled serving

Egg roll, 37 g net carbs per 1 large (¾" × 4" long) serving

Fish sticks, 18 g net carbs per 3 oz. serving

Flour tortilla, 15 g net carbs per 1 (8" in diameter) serving

French fries (homemade), 22 g net carbs per 17 medium-cut fry serving

Garbanzo beans, 13 g net carbs per ½ cup serving

Grilled cheese sandwich, 28 g net carbs per one sandwich serving

Hamburger with bun (plain), 26 g net carbs per ¼ lb. meat patty with medium-sized (40 gram) bun serving

Hot dog with bun (plain), 23 g net carbs per 1 (42 gram) link with 1 (40 gram) bun serving

Hot Pockets (ham and cheddar), 36 g net carbs per 1 (3.5 oz.) serving

Mashed potatoes, 31 g net carbs per 1 cup serving

Pasta, 41 g net carbs per 1 cup serving

Peanut-butter-and-jelly sandwich, 40 g net carbs per 1 sandwich serving

Pizza, 17 g net carbs per ⅛ slice thin-crust pizza (12" in diameter) serving

Quinoa, 35 g net carbs per 1 cup serving

Refried beans, 12 g net carbs per ½ cup serving

Sweet potato, 23 g net
   carbs per 1 medium-
   sized (2″×3″ long)
   serving
Tater Tots, 16 g net carbs
   per ½ cup serving

White rice, 44 g net carbs
   per 1 cup serving
Yams, 20 g net carbs
   per 1 medium-sized
   (2″×5″ long)
   serving

High-Carb Desserts

Apple pie, 52 g net carbs per
   ⅛ slice of double-crusted
   pie (9″ in diameter)
   serving
Brownie, 23 g net carbs
   per square (2″×2″)
   serving
Chips Ahoy! cookies, 21 g
   net carbs per 3 cookie
   serving
Chocolate (milk) bar, 31 g
   net carbs per 1 (56 gram)
   bar serving
Chocolate pudding (fat-free),
   27 g net carbs per ½ cup
   serving
Churros, 23 g net carbs
   per 2 (26 gram)
   serving
Cupcake (Hostess choco-
   late), 50 g net carbs per
   2 (45 gram) serving

Ice cream (vanilla), 24 g
   net carbs per ½ cup
   serving
Jell-O (with sugar), 19 g
   net carbs per ½ cup
   serving
M&M's (plain), 36 g net
   carbs per ¼ cup serving
M&M's (peanut), 27 g net
   carbs per ¼ cup serving
Oatmeal cookie, 20 g net
   carbs per 2 cookie (⅕″ in
   diameter) serving
Pecan pie (slice), 62 g net
   carbs per ⅛ slice of
   single-crust pie (9″ in
   diameter) serving
Pound cake, 46 g net carbs
   per slice (1″×5″×3″)
   serving
Sorbet (fruit), 34 g net carbs
   per ½ serving

High-Carb Drinks

Apple juice, 27 g net carbs per 8 fl. oz. serving

Beer, 13 g net carbs per 12 fl. oz. serving

Chocolate liqueur, 66 g net carbs per 4 fl. oz. serving

Coca-Cola (not diet), 35 g net carbs per 12 fl. oz. serving

Frappuccino chilled coffee drink (Starbucks), 53 g net carbs per 13.7 fl. oz. serving

Ginger ale (not diet), 36 g net carbs per 12 fl. oz. serving

Grape juice, 37 g net carbs per 8 fl. oz. serving

Horchata (rice), 27 g net carbs per 8 fl. oz. serving

Iced Caramel Macchiato (Starbucks), 37 g net carbs per 16 fl. oz. bottle serving

Iced Chai Tea Latte (Starbucks), 65 g net carbs per 24 fl. oz. (Venti) serving

Iced White Chocolate Mocha (Starbucks), 73 g net carbs per 24 fl. oz. (Venti) serving

Irish crème liqueur, 25 g net carbs per 4 fl. oz. serving

Jamba smoothie (Caribbean Passion), 98 g net carbs per 28 fl. oz. (large) serving

Jamba smoothie, (Mango-a-Go-Go), 119 g net carbs per 28 fl. oz. (large) serving

Lassi, 33 g net carbs per 1 cup serving

Margarita (mix), 28 g net carbs per 4 fl. oz. serving

Milk (2%), 12 g net carbs per 1 cup serving

Milk (nonfat), 12 g net carbs per 1 cup serving

Milk (skim or 1%), 12 g net carbs per 1 cup serving

Milk (whole), 12 g net carbs per 1 cup serving

Milkshake, vanilla shake (McDonald's), 131 g net carbs per 22 fl. oz. (large) serving

Mocha, 27 g net carbs per 8 fl. oz. serving

Mountain Dew, not diet, 46 g net carbs per 12 fl. oz. (can) serving

Pepsi, not diet, 41 g net carbs per 12 fl. oz. (can) serving

Piña colada (mix), 53 g net carbs per 4 fl. oz. serving

Pumpkin Spice Latte (Starbucks), 66 g net carbs per 20 fl. oz. (Venti) serving

Root beer, not diet, 47 g net carbs per 12 fl. oz. (can) serving

Soda, not diet, 35–47 g net carbs per 12 fl. oz. (can) serving

Sports drink, not diet, 16 g net carbs per 8 fl. oz. serving

Sprite, not diet, 38 g net carbs per 12 fl. oz. (can) serving

Sweet tea, not diet (McDonald's), 38 g net carbs per 32 fl. oz. (large) serving

Tea with honey, 17 g net carbs per 8 fl. oz. of steeped water with 1 tablespoon honey serving

Whiskey (cinnamon-flavored), 27 g net carbs per 1.5 fl. oz. serving

Wine cooler, varies per brand, estimated 20–41 g net carbs per 12 fl. oz. serving

What Should I Eat, Then?

Transitioning away from high-carb foods did not happen overnight for me. It might be hard for you to even imagine how I drastically reduced my daily net carbs intake from 1,000 grams of carbs a day down to a range of 20–50 grams. You might be curious about what kinds of foods I actually eat. Let me assure you that DIRTY, LAZY, KETO includes a ton of terrific choices that will keep you full all day long.

What does 20–50 grams of net carbs per day look like? I have enclosed my very official, patented DIRTY, LAZY,

KETO food pyramid to help you visualize my recommended way to spread out your carbs for a variety of satisfying foods (which I drew on the back of a napkin at the beginning of all of this). I sent this to the FDA for consideration to add to the sides of cereal boxes, but I have yet to hear back from them. *Yes, I'm joking, people!* The pyramid does not spell out what you HAVE to eat. I don't like a lot of rules, myself, so that part was important to me. Rather, I analyzed what I was eating (which has been quite effective, yes?), and mapped out in a visual way how I was eating. We will be going into this later in much more detail, but I'd like to give you a brief overview now so you don't skip ahead!

The top of the pyramid is the smallest category. This means I recommend eating just a handful of fruits, nuts, or seeds on any given day. Next is tier two, full-fat dairy. I encourage using common sense here, limiting how much dairy you eat because dairy is calorie dense and easy to overdo. Tier three represents nightshade vegetables, a category of vegetables you might be surprised to learn are higher in carbs. Lastly, tier four is where you can eat to your heart's content: non-starchy vegetables! Complemented with healthy fats and quality meats, this unique blend of foods represents the bulk of your weight-loss menu.

Everyone starts differently on DIRTY, LAZY, KETO. Some start cold turkey, drastically reducing all at once the amount of carbs they eat. Others prefer a slow, gradual transition period, taking a few weeks to ease into this new lifestyle. *Either way works!* There is no right or wrong way, only what works best for you.

Some of us have more weight to lose than others. Because of that variability, you are likely going to have to experiment with the number of net carbs you can eat while still losing weight. If you are starting at a higher weight, like I did, of close to three hundred pounds, you might get away with eating 50 grams of net carbs per day while still losing weight; lucky you! Score one for the big girls and boys. Conversely, those with less to lose might have to eat fewer carbs per day to see immediate results. If you're closer to goal weight, you might see better results by eating fewer net carbs, such as 20 grams per day.

Common sense needs to play a role here when determining how many net carbs per day to eat. You have to be realistic. There are internal and external factors influencing your weight loss, only some of which are in your control, including:

Activity level: The more active you are, the more you can eat and still lose weight.

Age: As we age, the speed of weight loss slows down.

Gender: Men generally lose weight faster than women because of higher testosterone levels and higher muscle mass.

Hormone Challenges: Menopause or thyroid imbalances might make weight loss trickier.

Current Weight: The amount of net carbs you eat will change as you lose weight.

Folks that have less weight to lose, or who are inactive, will likely need to consume fewer carbs per day to lose weight (closer to the 20 grams of net carbs per day). Conversely, superactive people can lose weight while eating more net carbs (eating as many as 50 grams of net carbs per day). Despite what other people say, finding the "perfect number of carbs" to eat is *not* an exact science! There is no magic calculator that can spit out this number. It's a moving target, too. As you lose weight, the number or range of net carbs you found once worked might need adjusting.

Whatever target (or range) you choose, be aware **there will always be a minimum number of carbs you must eat each day.** I rarely issue edicts like this, but I want you to be healthy, first and foremost, not just to lose weight. *Less is not always more.* Since the beginning of time, dieters have tried to figure out shortcuts for weight loss, I know. But trying to cut your carb spending below 20 grams of net carbs means you are not eating your vegetables, and you know how I feel about that!

We are all in such a hurry to lose weight, I get it. I'm sure you've heard of people trying to "game the system" by eating a zero-carb diet of let's say, all eggs, or only beef and butter. First of all, eating eggs all day just sounds GROSS! Can you imagine the gas and constipation? And, second, this kind of metabolic forced change is not healthy for your body. It's taxing on your kidneys and demoralizing to your self-esteem. Before you go defrosting pounds of ground round, please stop and think this through. This is where common sense needs to come into play.

Your goal is healthy, long-term weight loss, right? Not just a quick fix that lasts only while you can tolerate eating beef and butter.

Personally, I felt empowered eating within a range of 20–50 grams of net carbs per day. I liked the flexibility it gave me to eat out, enjoy a variety of real foods, and, most important, still feel like a "normal person" (*whoever that is*).

How you "spend your carbs" is up to you, but I would like to offer you some advice from the trenches.

Yes, you can spend your 20–50 grams of net carbs on crappy, "nutrition-less" food choices that taste good in the moment (pretty much anything in a box, can, bar, or pouch), but ultimately, poor choices catch up to you. What am I talking about here? Protein bars coated in fake chocolate, low-carb ice cream, keto-friendly chips—pretty much everything you ate "before" can now be bought for a pretty penny à la "keto-friendly" on Amazon. Sadly, none of these substitution choices will ever really fill you up.

Do I ever eat these instant foods from a box, can, pouch, or bar? Why, YES, I DO! This is DIRTY, LAZY, KETO, after all. The difference is that I don't eat these snacks *all the time*. I consider keto junk food to be "treats" or "emergency foods." These foods don't make up my entire menu. I'm not militant against keto junk food, as I eat this stuff, too, sometimes. I know that my secret success in losing so much weight is that *I don't rely on processed foods all day long like I used to*. Most of my meals *now* consist of eating *real* food, like meat, cheese, eggs, vegetables, nuts, and some fruits. I don't want to scare you off by suggesting you'll never eat chips again; that's not what I'm saying at all. I just want to show you what the end-game might look like. You can still have chips, but you likely won't want them once you get used to this new lifestyle.

Aside from sassiness, you will immediately notice that the principles of DIRTY, LAZY, KETO (created by yours truly) are completely different from keto diets you may have read about. Let's highlight a few key differences:

- Eating within **a range of net carbs** (as opposed to an exact number) will help you be more successful.
- There is no magic number for eating net carbs to lose weight. Everyone is different.
- If a food is important to you, find a way to still enjoy it.
- The possible effects of sugar substitutes are probably better for you than the complications of obesity.
- Use fat as a lever to make healthy food taste better, not as a macro goal.
- Keto junk food may be enjoyed once in a while, not all the time.
- Use common sense about eating too much dairy, especially HWC (heavy whipping cream) and cheese.
- Drink a lot of water. Have a diet soda. Drink a low-carb beer or cocktail when you want to. *(Ooooh, that should go first!)*
- Enjoy low-sugar fruit sometimes. *(This isn't Atkin's, people!)*
- You can eat lots (and lots) of non-starchy vegetables! Some people don't even "count" them in their daily carb allowance and still lose weight.
- DIRTY, LAZY, KETO is a lifestyle (not a temporary diet).

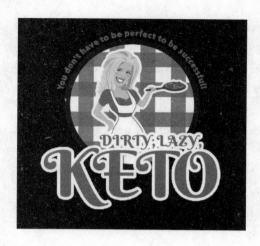

Eat Your Watermelon Already

Unlike other more rigid keto programs, DIRTY, LAZY, KETO is flexible to meet your needs. I once had a lady tell me she couldn't "do keto" because she likes to eat watermelon. First of all, I thought that was the weirdest reason ever: Who likes watermelon that much? (I kept *that* opinion to myself, though.) Instead, I responded *ever so suspiciously,* "Well, what if you just ate *some* watermelon?"

She looked at me dumbfounded, like I was completely off my rocker.

"But then I won't be in KETOSIS!" she screamed.

SO WHAT? I thought, sticking out my bottom lip to suppress crinkling my nose. I didn't say those words out loud, *trying to be respectful and all,* but on the inside, I was mystified. What was happening with this melon lover? It seemed she was more concerned with following the "rules" of keto than with actually losing weight. *Huh!* Hearing her truth brought on a *"watermelon moment"* for me, a big whopper of an "AHA!"

"You don't have to be perfect to be successful!"

#BreakTheRules

This conversation led me to create a personal motto: "You don't have to be perfect to be successful!" Yes, I'm breaking all the rules by telling you this little secret, but this is the truth. A bite of watermelon (or whatever forbidden food you just can't live without) isn't going to make or break your weight-loss efforts. Wrap your head around that statement and come back to me later, okay? If a food is important to you, find a way to enjoy it. Eat a little bit of it, or create a keto substitute, but, for cryin' out loud, don't ignore the fact that it's important to you. **Don't let the "watermelon" stop you from changing your life.**

TYPICAL MEALS ON DIRTY, LAZY, KETO

What does a typical meal look like on DIRTY, LAZY, KETO? The beauty of this lifestyle is the variety. It's hard to pinpoint what everyone's meals *should* look like, as there is no "right" or "wrong" meal. I can share, however, popular meals many people eat (including me), which might help you get started.

Breakfast

What's for breakfast? Eggs, bacon, or both—why not? Have you ever imagined a life where you can eat bacon and still lose weight? DIRTY, LAZY, KETO has arrived. Can I get an "amen," brothers and sisters?

In addition to using real butter in which to scramble your eggs, I recommend sneaking in some vegetables to your frying pan. Adding vegetables to breakfast starts the day off on the right note. Toss spinach, for example, into your omelet, egg bites, or smoothie.* Why am I suggesting eating vegetables and fat so early in the morning; am I touched or something? In addition to the health benefits provided, like vitamins and minerals (boring), the fiber in vegetables and fat from the butter will help you stay fuller for longer and even help you eat less during the actual meal. Now *that's* exciting, right?

I think of vegetables as necessary "filler" to slow down my eating.

If a hot breakfast isn't your style, maybe you would prefer creamy 5 percent fat yogurt or 4 percent milkfat cottage cheese? As long as you're not reaching for toast, cereal, or oats, you can be creative in your new morning routine. Who says you can't enjoy ham and cheese roll-ups for breakfast? Or how about an avocado?

Front-Loading versus Back-Loading

Because I exercise first thing in the morning, I like to front-load my carbs for the day. This means my breakfast meal is heavier in net carbs than, say, my dinner. I need that extra "oomph" to hit my blood sugar to get me going before I head to the gym or go on a run. I also find that by "spending" a large amount of carbs first thing, I feel more energized

---

* Recipes found in *The DIRTY, LAZY, KETO Cookbook: Bend the Rules to Lose the Weight!*

to take on the day. You will have to see what works best for your personality type and activity level.

Be aware that "saving" your carbs for later can sometimes backfire. I hear about dieters practically starving themselves all day in order to enjoy them at night, when they prefer to snack. The danger in back-loading your net carb spend is that by the time the "planned" eating window rolls around, you might be so hungry that you go completely overboard, like on a binge. Additionally, eating so many calories later in the day doesn't give you much opportunity to burn them off. If you eat late at night but then jump into bed for a long night's sleep, those carbs sit idly in your digestive system (or get stored as fat). Again, there are no rules here about how to enjoy your net carbs. I am just giving you some food for thought. Do what's best for you!

What can you drink in the morning? I would love for you to start drinking water, water, water, water, water—but of course you'll need some coffee first! YES, COFFEE IS OKAY!

A common question I hear from beginners is:

"What is bulletproof coffee, and do I have to drink that?"

The simple answer is no, you don't have to eat or drink anything weird. But you might feel like one of the cool kids after making a cup. I'll tell you a little more about this keto rite of passage.

Bulletproof Coffee (BPC)

BPC is just a fancy term for regular coffee with some fat in it. You will still lose weight *without* bulletproof coffee—or any coffee, for that matter! But for the sake of argument, let's take a look at what it is and why so many people swear by it.

Fat, as we know, is satiating and curbs hunger. Because bulletproof coffee includes fat, some espouse that it provides mental clarity and even starts their day with a clean boost. They believe that simply by changing your morning coffee from black coffee to adding fat also helps prolong the eating of their first meal of the day. You see, many try to "fast" as long as possible between their last meal at night and the first meal in the morning to assist with weight loss. Fat added to your morning coffee curbs your appetite, allowing you to "break the fast" with breakfast a bit later in the day. Bulletproof coffee is not a rule of DIRTY, LAZY, KETO. It's simply a tool you might find helpful (and maybe even fun).

Popular Bulletproof Coffee Additives

Unsalted butter: Kerrygold brand is popular, but let's be honest here: any unsalted butter will do, unless you have an incredible palate. Kerrygold brand butter is made from the cream of grass-fed Irish cows, *so apparently that must taste better.* Whether due to its high-quality cream or perhaps due to the current keto craze, Kerrygold brand butter is currently the third-bestselling butter in America. It's sold at Walmart,

Costco, and other major retailers. Butter offers 0 grams of net carbs per 1 tablespoon serving.

Ghee: Clarified butter, popular in Indian cooking, is an alternative ingredient to help add fat, but not a strong flavor, to your coffee. Ghee has 0 grams of net carbs per 1 tablespoon serving.

Heavy whipping cream (or whipping cream): is a liquid cream sold next to milk in the dairy section. In my opinion, you can substitute half-and-half for HWC, as it's more affordable and easier to find. I think it tastes pretty much the same when added to a cup of coffee—creamy and delicious! Notably, both heavy whipping cream and half-and-half are easy to overpour. A little goes a long way! The net carbs for both creams are pretty similar. Half-and-half has 1 gram of net carbs per 2 tablespoon serving (technically 1.4 grams of carbs, but that's *rounded down* on U.S. nutrition labels). Compare that to HWC, which has 1 gram of net carb per 1 tablespoon (again, technically it has .8 grams of carbs, but that's *rounded up* on U.S. nutrition labels).

Coconut milk: Canned, premium unsweetened coconut milk with 12–14% coconut fat provides an exotic, silky effect to brewed coffee and is thicker than comparable options. Depending on the brand, coconut milk has 0–1 gram of net carbs per 2.7 fl. oz. or ⅓ cup serving.

MCT oil: "MCT" stands for medium-chain triglyceride. (A commercial source would be coconut oil or palm-kernel oil.) This tasteless and odorless oil has been used historically as a fat source in infant formulas and more recently consumed by athletes and those looking for alternative energy sources. MCT oil is easily metabolized, bypassing the intestines for digestion, and heads straight to the liver. Some argue that MCT oil provides increased energy and aids in leading the body toward ketosis, the fat-burning state. Side effects of digesting MCT oil might include light-headedness, increased heart rate, and diarrhea, so use with caution. *Less is more* when it comes to MCT oil. Its power is not just limited to your guts; my friend Carol reported that MCT oil added to her Styrofoam coffee cup caused it to literally explode in her hands. *I'm not joking!* MCT Oil has 0 grams of net carbs per tablespoon serving.

Sweeteners: Can you add sugar-free sweeteners to your coffee? Die-hard strict ketogenic followers argue against artificial sugars of any kind; they claim that the use of artificial sweeteners will wreak havoc on your blood sugar and derail weight-loss success. Alternatively, some folks avoid sugar-free sweeteners due to their potential health risks. Personally, I believe adding artificial sweeteners to coffee (or anywhere else!) is a personal choice, not a "rule" about something you *can or cannot eat*. Net carbs vary according to brand of sweetener; usually, sugar-free sweeteners range from 0–1 net carb per packet or gram.

Personally, I had a hard time changing my coffee routine. I was used to "real-deal" milk and sugar in my coffee and I didn't want to let go of that sweet flavor. For years, I relied on sugar-free coffee creamers for my morning kick start. Nestlé Coffee mate Sugar-free French Vanilla, Hazelnut, and Italian Sweet Crème were my favorites. Flavored creamers range from 0 to 3 grams of net carb per tablespoon serving, depending on brand. When those weren't available, I would use half-and-half with a splash of Torani or DaVinci flavored sugar-free syrups, which range from 0 to 1 gram of net carbs per tablespoon depending on flavor and brand. (Note: Many sugar-free syrups are available at Starbucks and even McDonald's!*) This is your body, and you get to decide whether or not to supplement your coffee. Artificial flavors, coloring, or sweeteners are allowed. DIRTY, LAZY, KETO has your back if someone wants to call in the keto police for a throwdown.

It's almost comical how strongly we feel about our morning coffee. Ask any keto dieter his or her opinion on the matter and you most certainly will get an earful! The bottom line is that bulletproof coffee is a personal choice. Fat added to coffee is a means to help control your blood sugar and prevent overeating later. (It's *not* a magic potion that guarantees weight loss.) Think of bulletproof coffee as an option, not a requirement, in your DIRTY, LAZY, KETO lifestyle.

Lunch and Dinner

I'm going to speak very generally here, but most of your DIRTY, LAZY, KETO non-breakfast meals will consist of some quality protein, healthy fats, and lots of non-starchy vegetables. You can mix and match combinations of the three with endless possibilities. Googling recipes or exploring sites like Pinterest will undoubtedly provide you with millions of free meal ideas. But will these recipes meet your

---

* To help support your decisions at coffee and fast-food restaurants, I created with William Laska, *DIRTY, LAZY, KETO Fast Food Guide: 10 Carbs or Less* (Amazon, 2018).

needs? It's been my experience that keto recipe sites are hard to use. They are often riddled with click-bait advertisements hovering over the recipe's directions. To make matters worse, many recipes are ridiculously high in net carbs, or lack nutrition information altogether.

It's definitely the wild west out there in keto-land. Because online recipes aren't regulated, be sure to *calculate the macros* yourself for recipes before preheating the oven. Your expectations of what constitutes a low-carb recipe might be *very different* from someone else's! I have stumbled across many so-called "keto" recipes that have as many as 40 carbs *per serving*! It's absolutely maddening. To help make cooking easier for you, I've published *The DIRTY, LAZY, KETO Cookbook: Bend the Rules to Lose the Weight!** which contains 100 delicious easy-to-make recipes *all less than 10 net carbs per serving*—that's right, all less than 10 net carbs! For those on an especially tight budget, also be on the lookout for my next book, *The DIRTY, LAZY, KETO Dirt Cheap Cookbook*†.

Tips to Make Meals Easy

In the beginning, you might find it helpful to stick to a few dinners that "work for you." You may want to jump-start your confidence by first having some success on the scale before branching out to trying more complex recipes. It's okay to repeat meals and add more variety later once you get

---

* Simon & Schuster, 2020
† Simon & Schuster, 2020

your footing. Keep things simple so you don't become over-whelmed. This is your dance, my friend, so you get to choose the steps. Start off slowly.

To make planning easier for you, think about it this way: pick a protein, a vegetable, and a fat.

Here are some simple ideas to get you going:

- Chicken with a green salad and dressing
- Beef and broccoli stir-fry with oil
- Salmon and asparagus with butter
- Pork chop with green beans and almonds
- Omelet with spinach and feta cheese
- Lettuce-wrapped deli meat with cheese, mayo, and vegetable
- Roast turkey breast with mashed cauliflower and gravy
- Shrimp with alfredo sauce over zucchini "zoodles"

It's tempting when first starting DIRTY, LAZY, KETO to think that you "must have" expensive keto substitution items. You might naïvely assume that because an item says "keto" at the grocery store, you need to buy it. WRONG! Here is an example: Everyone loves pizza, right? Some snazzy marketing guy figured out there must be a demand for low-carb pizza crust. He reconfigured a recipe that substituted cauliflower for white flour and is now making a boatload of money selling these crust alternatives at Target and Costco. Do you have to buy these and other "substitution items"? NO, YOU DO NOT. You might even be disappointed at the net carb count per slice. *Read the nutrition labels!* Remember, just because it says "keto" on the label doesn't mean it's low enough in carbs to meet your standards.

I consider these substitutions to be luxury items. I rarely used high-priced packaged alternatives, and I still lost weight. Can you buy them if your budget allows you to? YES, YOU CAN! In my opinion, they aren't necessary, but can be "helpful" if used appropriately. Let me explain.

There are a lot of changes in front of you. It's hard to let go of old habits. I understand—I've been there. My family ate pizza every Friday night for, like, one hundred years, so when I realized I had to say goodbye to that tradition, I felt left out and *a bit resentful,* if I'm being totally honest. Buying one of these pizza substitute crusts might have helped me temporarily, but in the end, I needed to develop a new routine for my Friday night that was sustainable. I learned that I didn't need to eat pizza to take part in the Friday night tradition. Spending time with my loved ones was really what mattered, not the food. Do you see where I'm going with this?

I found chicken wings, a salad, and a low-carb beer was an easy substitution for Friday-night pizza. Oh, and focusing on my family, rather than the food!

Expensive specialty keto foods will ultimately let you down with taste, availability, and price. I would like to reiterate how the retail substitution (like keto pizzas) are a "crutch" to help transition eating habits from "old" to the "new" behaviors. They are certainly "allowed" on DIRTY, LAZY, KETO, but I urge you to start thinking of new ways to meet your needs permanently. **Time spent with family and friends will leave you more satisfied than a pizza ever will.**

Friday-Night Wings with Bing-Bang Sauce

Yield: 3 servings 〉 Prep time: 15 minutes 〉 Cook time: 50 minutes 〉 5 net carbs/serving

Friday nights have always been a zoo at our house. The kids would invite their friends over, and we would all share pizza. In the summer, my husband and I would supervise from our lawn chairs set inside a baby pool and drink cold beer with our slices while the kids played with water balloons. A few things have changed since then: now I'm eating chicken wings, drinking a low-carb beer, but wearing a bikini!

INGREDIENTS

½ cup unblanched almond flour (super-fine)

½ cup grated Parmesan cheese

2 tablespoons baking powder

4 tablespoons hemp hearts (you may substitute crushed pork rinds)

¼ (1-oz.) package ranch-seasoning powder

2 large eggs, beaten

1 tablespoon (full-fat) half-and-half

nonstick cooking spray

2½ pounds (about 18) chicken wings, trimmed

Bing-Bang Sauce

½ cup (full-fat) mayonnaise

2 packets of zero-carbs sweetener

1 teaspoon sriracha sauce

1 teaspoon vinegar (plain white distilled or apple cider vinegar, your choice)

⅛ teaspoon soy sauce

1 celery stalk, trimmed and cut into 4-inch sections

DIRECTIONS

1. Preheat oven to 425°F.
2. In a small bowl, mix dry ingredients (except sweetener). Set aside.
3. In a separate small bowl, whisk eggs with half-and-half.
4. Line an extra-large baking sheet with foil. Set wire rack inside baking sheet. Spray with nonstick cooking spray.
5. Don plastic gloves, if desired. Assign one hand for dipping chicken in egg bath (step 1), and the other for rolling wings in dry rub (step 2). Complete breading task until all wings are covered.
6. Spread out wings on wire rack without letting them touch.
7. Bake 25 minutes. Turn wings over gently, being careful not to loosen coating.
8. Return to oven and bake 25 minutes longer.
9. While wings are cooking, make Bing-Bang Sauce for dipping.
10. In a small bowl, combine mayo, sugar substitute, sriracha, vinegar, and soy sauce.
11. Serve chicken wings warm with Bing-Bang Sauce on the side with cut celery. Best enjoyed with a low-carb beer!

Dumpster Salad with Green-Machine Dressing

Yield: 2 serving 〉 Prep time: 10 minutes 〉 Cook time: 0 minutes 〉
8 net carbs/serving

Since eating helps me relax, I prefer recipes with large serving sizes. I want the food (and relaxation) to last as long as possible! Dumpster Salad is my way of using every healthy ingredient in my produce drawer. It's filling, healthy, and delicious when topped with my favorite creamy homemade salad dressing. Plus, I get to eat a humongous bowl of food!

INGREDIENTS

4 cups romaine salad mix

2 large hard-boiled eggs, peeled and sliced

½ small tomato, chopped

2 tablespoons sliced red onion

1 cup raw broccoli florets

1 cup raw cauliflower florets

½ cup diced unpeeled cucumber

¼ cup sliced mushrooms

4 oz. cooked chicken breast

½ cup crumbled (full-fat) feta cheese

1 tablespoon shelled sunflower seeds

6 slices cooked turkey bacon, crumbled

Green-Machine Dressing

¼ cup full-fat mayonnaise

¼ cup full-fat sour cream

1 large ripe avocado, seeded, peeled, and mashed

2 tablespoons lime juice

2 tablespoons water

⅛ teaspoon salt

DIRECTIONS

1. In a small bowl, thoroughly whisk all dressing ingredients well. Set aside.
2. In large salad bowl, combine all vegetables. Divide evenly into two serving bowls. Top with equal amounts of chicken, cheese, sunflower seeds, and bacon.
3. Serve with Green-Machine Dressing.

Dessert

While desserts are definitely not a meal, many of us with a history of being overweight have treated dessert like an all-you-can-eat buffet. You are not alone with your sweet tooth, my friend! Physical cravings for sugar will diminish over time with DIRTY, LAZY, KETO, sure, but until we eliminate emotional triggers that scream "SUGAR . . . NOW!" there will always be a need for something sweet.

There is no judgment here. I come from a generation of eating Fruit Loops and drinking Kool-Aid, so clearly my blood runs thick with artificial colors and flavorings.

Using artificial sweeteners (or natural sugar substitutes) is a personal choice. There are many to choose from, and I'm sure some are healthier than others. I'm not here to advocate which one you choose (if any), but I am going to climb on my soapbox and scream to all the members listening in keto-land, "GO AHEAD AND ENJOY YOUR KETO-FRIENDLY DESSERT!"

Some people get all riled up about this topic. They have VERY STRONG FEELINGS and will begin SHOUTING about their sugar belief systems. I am so curious about this. Why do folks care if I put Splenda in my coleslaw? *I mean, really!* I agree with the overall concept that sprinkling chemicals (or natural monk fruit, *whatever*) on my food might not be the best idea, but if I need that crutch to be successful at losing weight and improving my overall health for the "big picture," then why isn't that okay?

There are a few things happening here that I would like to point out. First of all, I would like to question the motives of the "keto police." If a critic honestly has my best interest in mind, then stop me now and let me thank that person. Not everyone is trying to be supportive, however. Some people like to criticize others because they are desperately *trying to feel better about themselves.* They are trying to prop themselves up onto a righteous high horse to create false feelings of superiority. I suspect that they are sad underneath their smugness; I have to believe that they are struggling just like the rest of us. But aside from their motives, let me defend those of us who continue to indulge in sugar-free treats. There is no shame in wanting something sweet. We are not weak for desiring pleasure!

Can I stop and restate the obvious here?

"I KNOW THIS FAKE-SUGAR CRAP ISN'T GOOD FOR ME, BUT RIGHT NOW I NEED IT TO PREVENT ME FROM GIVING UP."

All that being said, I will leave you with one final thought about sugar substitutions, natural or artificial, and those that fall somewhere in between. Even if they are low-carb or altogether sugar-free, some products can trigger your blood sugar to rise and, unfortunately, activate your sugar-craving cycle. *This is so not fair!* For example, I can't ever eat just one piece of sugar-free gum. I pop one piece after another into my mouth (in rapid succession), until I either run out of gum or irritate whoever is with me with all my chomping noises. I just *can't get enough* of that sugary explosion in my mouth. It's a little embarrassing, I know!

Everyone reacts to sugar substitutes differently, and only you can determine if sweeteners are helpful or harmful to your weight-loss success. If you find that eating something with one of these substitutions causes you to fall back into "old patterns," then perhaps you may want to avoid that substitute in the future or limit its quantity. I know myself pretty well, and I have trouble with portion control, especially around baked goods. Even if a dessert is created from a low-carb recipe, I will go completely overboard. I will lick the spatula, eat most of the batter from the bowl, and then cut piece after piece of a finished dessert until it's gone. *Yep, I'm classy like that!*

Sugar Substitutes

Have you heard that the herb cilantro tastes like soap to some people? I'm not kidding. Some kind of taste bud miscommunication occurs between the tongue and the brain and instead of tasting a breezy, fresh herb, they want to hurl. These disadvantaged souls will never enjoy guacamole the way I do. The way people experience sugar substitutes is pretty similar. The reactions are all over the place! One person's favorite is spit out in disgust by another. It's become evident to me just *how personal a decision* it is to find a sugar substitute you can tolerate.

None of these, I repeat, NOT A ONE will taste *exactly* like sugar. You must *adjust* your expectations. To make your selection even more complicated, you may find they taste differently after heated or cooked in baked goods.

Additionally, we all have different comfort levels about consuming artificially processed or chemically created ingredients. Choosing a more natural product might be important to you at the expense of taste, or even cost. Perhaps safety is your number one concern, and you trust a brand that has been on the market for a longer period of time. All of your concerns are valid. I support whatever sugar substitute you are most comfortable with. Expect to experiment before finding the best fit *for you*.

I wish I could make this easier for you, but in my opinion, there is no universal front runner. Choosing a sugar substitute is a matter of your personal preference. I will quickly summarize available popular options.*

---

* Leading brands included (not a complete list).

Brand Name	Type	Approved	Net Carbs/serving*
Equal	Aspartame	1981	>1 g net carb per 1 packet
Lakanto	Swingle Fruit*	Pending**	0 g net carbs per 1 teaspoon
Monk Fruit	Swingle Fruit*	Pending**	0 g net carb per 1 packet
Monk Fruit in the Raw	Swingle Fruit*	Pending**	0 g net carb per 1 packet
Necta Sweet	Saccharin	1958	1 g net carb per 1 packet
Nevella	Sucralose	1999	>1 g net carb per 1 packet
NutraSweet	Aspartame	1981	>1 g net carb per 1 packet
Pure Fruit	Swingle Fruit*	Pending**	0 g net carb per 1 packet
Pure Stevia	Stevia plant-based	Pending**	1 g net carb per 1 packet
PureLo	Swingle Fruit*	Pending**	0 g net carbs per teaspoon
Pure Monk	Swingle Fruit*	Pending**	0 g net carbs per teaspoon
PureVia	Stevia plant-based	Pending**	1 g net carb per 1 packet
Splenda	Sucralose	1999	1 g net carb per 1 packet
Sugar Twin	Aspartame	1981	>1 g net carb per 1 packet
Sunett	Ace-K†	1988	0 g net carbs per 1 packet
Swanson PureLo	Swingle Fruit*	Pending**	0 g net carb per 1 packet
Sweet Leaf	Stevia plant-based	Pending**	1 g net carb per 1 packet
Sweet One	Ace-K†	1988	0 g net carbs per 1 packet
Sweet Twin	Saccharin	1958	1 g net carb per 1 packet
Sweet'N Low	Saccharin	1958	1 g net carb per 1 packet
Swerve	Swingle Fruit*	Pending**	0 g net carbs per 1 teaspoon
Truvia	Stevia plant-based	Pending**	1 g net carb per 1 packet
Zing	Stevia plant-based	Pending**	1 g net carb per 1 packet

* Swingle fruit extract, also known as Monk Fruit or Luo Han Guo.

†Acesulfame-K

** GRAS statement issued for specific uses. Approval pending. www.fda.gov/food/food-additives-petitions/additional-information-about-high-intensity-sweeteners-permitted-use-food-united-states

---

* Serving sizes of artificial sweeteners may vary because of product potency.

According to the chart, all of the sugar substitutes appear to have a similar net carb count per serving—0 or 1 gram of net carbs per one packet or one teaspoon serving. This small serving size can be deceiving. Since U.S. nutrition labels round nutrients up or down to the nearest whole number, this leads to confusion when the serving size is increased for baking. Let's take Splenda, for example. A 1-gram packet of Splenda has less than 1 net carb per serving according to the package nutrition label. Well that sounds pretty great? *Not so fast.* What happens when I use Splenda to make my infamous Birthday Cheesecake* recipe, which calls for 1¼ cups artificial sweetener? How does Splenda measure up then?

According to the Splenda for professionals website (why this information is only available to professionals, I don't know)† there are 22 grams of net carbohydrates per cup of Splenda. If I use Splenda in my Birthday Cheesecake recipe, I'm adding 28 grams of net carbs to my dessert! (In case I went too fast for ya there, 1.25 cups × 22 grams = 27.5, which is rounded up to 28 grams of net carbs). *That's just upsetting.*

Are there any other options? A new hybrid of artificial sweeteners is emerging that blend artificial sweeteners with sugar alcohols (such as erythritol). Because sugar alcohols are not digested, these carbohydrates are subtracted from the total number of carbohydrates per serving, lowering the overall remaining amount of net carbs (review the "How to Read a Nutrition Label," p. 00, if needed). Let's apply this knowledge to a second example with Lakanto Monkfruit Sweet-

---

* *The DIRTY, LAZY, KETO Cookbook: Bend the Rules to Lose the Weight!* (Simon & Schuster, 2020).
† https://www.splendaprofessional.com/studies-science/splenda-sweeteners-compared-sugar

ener, which contains both erythritol and monk fruit extract. A serving size of 1 teaspoon yields 0 grams of net carbs (4 g of sugar alcohol subtracted from the total carbohydrate of 4 g per teaspoon resulting in 0 g of net carbs). But what happens when we pour a full cup? Surprisingly, the amount of net carbs stays the same—*zero*! Since there are 60 teaspoons in 1.25 cups, I multiply $0 \times 1.25 = 0$ grams of net carbs. *My Birthday Cheesecake sounds even better right now!*

The striking difference between the viable amount of net carbs isn't the only factor to be considered, however. Not everyone can tolerate sugar alcohols or artificial sweeteners. Some people experience uncomfortable side effects. Safety, taste, cost, manufacturing preference, and product availability must also be considered. Bottom line? There is no clear answer. Therefore, *use what you are most comfortable with.*

What About Flour?

For some reason, flour substitutes don't generate as much drama, despite their ability to negatively affect one's blood sugar. Perhaps this is because we don't usually "crave" flour in the same way we "crave" sugar. Or maybe it is because flour substitutes aren't riddled with chemicals as sugar substitutes often are. Whatever the reason, people seem more open-minded to swap out traditional white flour for something with fewer carbs. Flour substitutes vary in terms of carbs per serving, taste, and performance within a recipe, so do your research before replacing white flour in your food preparation. Coconut flour, for example, has a strong, nutty flavor, which comes through in recipes. You'll have to play around with the different options to discover what flour substitutes make the most sense in your recipes.

Flour Substitutes

Almond flour (super-fine), 3 g net carbs per ¼ cup serving

Carbquik Baking Mix, 2 g net carbs per ⅓ cup serving

Coconut flour, 4–5 net carbs per ¼ cup serving

Flaxseed (ground), 1 g net carb per 2 tablespoon serving

Flaxseed meal (whole), 2 g net carbs per 2½ tablespoon serving

Hemp seeds (shelled), 1 g net carbs per 3 tablespoon serving

Parmesan cheese, 0 g carb per 1 teaspoon serving

Pork rinds, 0 g net carbs per 1 oz. serving

Psyllium husk powder, 1 g net carb per 1 teaspoon serving

Soy flour, 5 g net carbs per ¼ cup serving

Vital wheat gluten flour, 1 g net carb per 1 tablespoon serving

White and Wheat Flour (for reference)

Only for reference, note that all-purpose enriched white flour has 84 g net carbs per 1 cup serving and all-natural whole-wheat flour follows close behind with 72 g net carbs per 1 cup serving.

Snacks

I exist in a constant state of anxiety and fear that I will find myself in an unexpected location without keto-friendly food. I also have irrational thoughts that a single hunger pang will lead to uncontrollable carbohydrate "binge eating."

**I definitely don't want my lack of planning
to be a reason for me to "fall off the wagon"
and end up snacking on a dozen churros!**

Because of my deep-seated fears, you will always find my purse stuffed with secret DIRTY, LAZY, KETO snacks. Some of my favorites are listed on the next two pages.

**To this day, my coworkers tease me about a time
we were traveling for work and the TSA inspector
identified and inspected "suspicious items"
in my carry-on luggage: Ziploc bags packed full
of turkey bacon, celery sticks, and avocados!**

Whether I'm driving across the country, sitting through a long meeting, or taking a walk around the block, I've been known to have an excessive amount of options to enjoy. Plan for success, people, even if it's embarrassing.

DIRTY, LAZY, KETO Snacks Ideas

- Avocado, 1 g net carbs per ⅓ of a medium (50 gram) avocado serving
- Bacon, 0 g net carbs for 2 fried slices (15 grams each) serving
- Brazil nuts, 1 g net carb per 1 oz. serving
- Celery, 1 g net carb per 1 cup or long stalk (11″ long) serving
- Cheese (string, cubed, sliced), 1 g net carb per 1 oz. serving
- Coconut (shredded, unsweetened), 2 g net carbs per 2 tablespoon serving
- Deli meat, 1 g net carb per 2 oz. serving
- Egg (hard-boiled),1 g net carb per large egg serving
- Gelatin (sugar-free), 0 g net carb per ½ cup
- Hazelnuts, 2 g net carbs per 1 oz. serving
- Jerky (original Slim Jim), 1 g net carb per stick (9.6 gram) serving
- Macadamia nuts, 2 g net carbs per 1 oz. serving
- Olives (black), 1 g net carb per 2 olive serving
- Pecan nuts (halves), 1 g net carbs per ¼ cup serving
- Pickles (dill), 1–2 g net carbs per ¾ spear (1 oz.) serving
- Pork rinds (original), 0 g net carb per .5 oz. (14 gram) serving
- Protein bar (Quest), 4 g net carbs per 1 (2.12 oz.) bar (60 gram) serving
- Seaweed snacks, 1 g net carb per 5 gram serving

- String cheese, 1 g net carb per 1 piece (28 gram) serving
- Tofu, 2 g net carbs per 3 oz. (1″ slice) serving
- Water, water, water, water! 0 g net carb
- Yogurt, 3–9 g net carbs (varies per brand) per 1 cup serving
- Zucchini (raw), 1 g net carb per 1 cup serving

Drinks

In addition to drinking your water, water, water, water, DIRTY, LAZY, KETO supports your decision to drink diet soda. *Gasp!* You can even enjoy alcohol that is low-carb or zero carbs. *WOW!* Again, best lifestyle EVER! Black coffee and tea contain zero carbs, too. Because your carbs are yours to spend, you might like almond milk (or other dairy-alternative milk) to slip into your smoothies. I like to focus on what I CAN HAVE and not what I CAN'T. I'm *not* going to focus on the long list of sugary beverages that have more carbs in one cup than I would eat in an entire day. Those drinks are a thing of the past. Instead, let's talk about sugar-free options:

DIRTY, LAZY, KETO Drink Ideas (Nonalcoholic)

Zero Net Carbs Drink Ideas (per 8 fl. oz. cup serving)

- Coffee (black), 0 g net carbs
- Diet soda, 0 g net carbs (check label to ensure you select a diet soda without any carbs)

- Electrolyte water (MiO, Powerade, Smartwater), 0 g net carbs
- Energy drinks, sugar-free (check the label, as some still contain carbs), 0 g net carbs
- Mineral water or naturally flavored water, 0 g net carbs
- Seltzer water (sugar-free), 0 g net carbs
- Soda water (sugar-free), 0 g net carbs
- Tea (herbal, black, green), 0 g net carbs
- Tonic water (sugar-free), 0 g net carbs
- Water, 0 g net carbs

Low Net Carbs Drink Ideas (per 8 fl. oz. cup serving)

- Bone broth, 1 g net carb per serving
- Citrus (from concentrate) added to water, 1–2 net carbs per teaspoon serving
- Coffee with sugar-free creamer, estimated 0–3 g net carbs per serving of coffee with 1 tablespoon creamer serving
- Dairy alternative drink (unsweetened almond, coconut, cashew, flaxseed, hemp, or soy milks), ranges between 0 and 2 g net carbs per serving
- Energy drinks (low-carb), ranges between 3 and 5 g net carbs per serving
- Protein smoothies, net carbs depend on ingredients chosen
- Vegetable smoothies, net carbs depend on ingredients chosen

Low Net Carbs Alcoholic Drink Ideas

Contrary to what you may have heard, it's still possible to stay in ketosis, or weight-loss mode, while drinking an ice cold, low-carb beer. True, there is no such thing as an official "keto beer," but there are many options on the market that can still fit into your DIRTY, LAZY, KETO lifestyle. Let's check out a few popular brands for comparison. Note that unlike popular websites that try to fool you with "per ounce" statistics and lots of decimal points, I am providing the rounded-up carb count for the *full bottle or can*. Who drinks just an ounce? Not me. Also, I want real numbers I can keep track of after having a beer, not a bunch of partial decimal points!

Lower Carb Beer and Malt Alcoholic Beverages

Net carbs are rounded to the nearest whole number for a 12 fl. oz. serving. *Drink responsibly.*

Low-Carb Beers

- Amstel Light, 5 g net carbs
- Bud Ice, 4 g net carbs
- Bud Light, 7 g net carbs
- Busch Light, 3 g net carbs
- Coors Light, 5 g net carbs
- Corona Light, 5 g net carbs
- Corona Premier, 3 g net carbs
- Keystone Light, 5 g net carbs

- Michelob Ultra, 3 g net carbs
- Miller Lite, 3 g net carbs
- Natural Light, 3 g net carbs

Low-Carb Malt Beverages*

- Bon & Viv Spiked Seltzer (Cape Cod Cranberry), 1 g net carbs
- Bon & Viv Spiked Seltzer (Indian River Grapefruit), 1 g net carbs
- Bon & Viv Spiked Seltzer (Valencia Orange), 1 g net carbs
- Bon & Viv Spiked Seltzer (West Indies Lime), 1 g net carbs
- Henry's Hard Sparkling Water (Blueberry Lemon), 3 g net carbs
- Henry's Hard Sparkling Water (Lemon Lime), 3 g net carbs
- Henry's Hard Sparkling Water (Strawberry Kiwi), 3 g net carbs
- Smirnoff Spiked Sparkling Seltzer (Berry Lemonade), 1 g net carbs
- Smirnoff Spiked Sparkling Seltzer (Cranberry Lime), 1 g net carbs
- Smirnoff Spiked Sparkling Seltzer (Piña Colada), 1 g net carbs
- Smirnoff Spiked Sparkling Seltzer (Piña Colada), 1 g net carbs

---

* As new flavors are introduced from these companies, be sure to look at the company's website directly for up-to-date nutritional information.

- Smirnoff Spiked Sparkling Seltzer (Piña Colada), 1 g net carbs
- Smirnoff Spiked Sparkling Seltzer (Raspberry Rose), 1 g net carbs
- The Shell House* Sparkling Hard Seltzer (Meyer Lemon) 5 g net carbs
- The Shell House Sparkling Hard Seltzer (Pomegranate) 5 g net carbs
- The Shell House Sparkling Hard Seltzer (Pomegranate) 5 g net carbs
- The Shell House Sparkling Hard Seltzer (Pomegranate) 5 g net carbs
- Truly Hard Seltzer (Black Cherry), 2 g net carbs
- Truly Hard Seltzer (Mango), 2 g net carbs
- Truly Hard Seltzer (Passion Fruit), 2 g net carbs
- Truly Hard Seltzer (Pineapple), 2 g net carbs
- Truly Hard Seltzer (Raspberry Lime), 2 g net carbs
- Truly Hard Seltzer (Watermelon and Kiwi), 2 g net carbs
- Truly Hard Seltzer (with a hint of Grapefruit), 2 g net carbs
- Truly Hard Seltzer (with a hint of Lemon), 2 g net carbs
- Truly Hard Seltzer (with a hint of Lime), 2 g net carbs
- Truly Hard Seltzer (with a hint of Orange), 2 g net carbs
- White Claw Hard Seltzer (Acai and Raspberry), 2 g net carbs

---

* The Shell House is a house brand sold only at Trader Joe's.

- White Claw Hard Seltzer (Black Cherry), 2 g net carbs
- White Claw Hard Seltzer (Blueberry), 2 g net carbs
- White Claw Hard Seltzer (Mango), 2 g net carbs
- White Claw Hard Seltzer (Natural Lime), 2 g net carbs
- White Claw Hard Seltzer (Raspberry), 2 g net carbs
- White Claw Hard Seltzer (Ruby Grapefruit), 2 g net carbs
- White Claw Hard Seltzer (Wild Berry), 2 g net carbs
- White Claw Pure Hard Seltzer (unflavored), 0 g net carbs
- Wild Basin Boozy Sparkling Water (Classic Lime), 1 g net carbs
- Wild Basin Boozy Sparkling Water (Cucumber Peach), 1 g net carbs
- Wild Basin Boozy Sparkling Water (Lemon Agave Hibiscus), 1 g net carbs
- Wild Basin Boozy Sparkling Water (Melon Basil), 1 g net carbs

Cocktail Hour

What about keto cocktails? As long as you choose a low-carb liquor or zero-carb hard alcohol, DIRTY, LAZY, KETO and cocktail hour coexist quite nicely. The problem isn't finding low-carb alcoholic drinks—there are plenty to choose from! The challenge lies in making the right decisions involving food after imbibing. Chips and dip? Bring it on! Want to order pizza? Why not? **DIRTY, LAZY, KETO and cocktails** harmonize as long as you can maintain self-control and avoid carby choices at the late-night drive-thru. Let's keep it real.

Keto alcohol options aren't just limited to low-carb beer. Create keto cocktails using low-carb liquor or no-carb hard alcohol. Mixed with a sugar-free energy drink or flavored sugar-free carbonated water, these concoctions will whet your whistle without causing a keto weight-loss stall. Prefer something sweeter? Mix your drink with sugar-free piña colada flavor, margarita mix, or flavored water packets. I keep an assortment of flavors in my kitchen (purchased from the Dollar Store, of all places!). Brands I often purchase include: Crush, Crystal Light, Dasani, Mio, Hawaiian Punch, Jolly Rancher, and Wyler's. Now that you have plenty of "mixer ideas," let's identify sugar-free spirits to add to your cocktail.

How many carbs are in clear hard alcohols, you might ask? All unflavored hard alcohol—vodka, gin, rum, tequila, and sake—contain zero carbs. Be sure to select traditional labels unadulterated by gimmicks. *No cotton candy or cupcake vodka tonight!* Prepare your cocktail by adding ice, water, and a sugar-free flavor packet. My favorite vodka mixer is Crush pineapple sugar-free powdered drink mix over ice with a splash of unsweetened coconut milk* for a Caribbean piña colada. *Cheers.*

What about whiskey and other dark spirits? I was surprised about their lack of carbs, too. Even though it's an amber-colored alcohol, whiskey still contains zero carbs. I sometimes get confused between the darker alcohols (maybe

---

* Coconut milk—canned, premium unsweetened coconut milk with 12–14% coconut fat has 1 g net carb per 2.7 oz. or ⅓ cup serving.

after having a glass or two?), but it helps to avoid, in general, all of the flavored alcohols that contain unnecessary sugar. Even dark hard **alcohols—whiskey, scotch, dark rum, brandy, cognac, and bourbon**—all have zero carbs. In general, avoid the heavily marketed "flavored" varieties which likely contain sugar. Pass on the cinnamon Fireball shots (38 grams of carbs) and order a straight-up whiskey.*

Does your keto cocktail feel stronger than it used to? You may have noticed that your alcohol tolerance has decreased since you started DIRTY, LAZY, KETO. This is because you have fewer carbs floating around to absorb the alcohol in your system (compared to before, when you ate more carbs). To counterbalance this effect, drink less alcohol, plan to eat more carbs when drinking, or switch to a drink with less potency. Instead of a mixed drink, enjoy a dirty keto alternative like wine. How many carbs are in wine, you may be wondering? What follows are some estimates. Note the provided net carbs here are per serving, which apparently is only 5 ounces! (*Who serves themselves only 5 ounces?!*)

Wine and DIRTY, LAZY, KETO

If you must enjoy a glass of wine, be sure to choose wisely. There can be a lot of hidden sugar in our favorite grape beverage! The key to choosing a wine with the least amount of carbs is the word "dry."

For some reason, everything to do with wine has to sound

---

* If you insist on a fireball shot, drop a sugar-free cinnamon candy into your shot of whiskey. Just because you follow DIRTY, LAZY, KETO doesn't mean you're a party pooper.

fancy. Vintners can't just say the word "dry" and make it easy for us! (Or even better, fess up and slap a nutrition label on the side of the bottle.) Because we are left in the dark, it's easy to get confused over exotic phrases printed on the wine bottle. Most people don't know that a Riesling or Muscat is a syrupy-sweet dessert wine, or that "brut" means dry— equating to less sugar. Instead of guessing, use this guide to help you make an educated decision. Don't be afraid to ask the waiter, bartender (or sommelier, if you're super-fancy!) for a recommendation, too.

As I mentioned before when talking about beer, I prefer to round up (or down) when counting carbs in alcoholic drinks. I don't know about you, but even after a sip of alcohol my math skills go out the window. Let's keep this simple! The provided list of wines are rounded to the nearest number, and based on a *5-ounce serving*. I have to admit, I was surprised at the number of DIRTY, LAZY, KETO options for both white and red wines. Because everyone has different tastes and varying comfort levels with the amount of carbs they consume, I have included a wide range of options here. *Drink responsibly.*

White Wine Recommendations (5 oz. serving)

- Champagne, 1 g net carbs
- Wine spritzer (your choice of dry wine from list below diluted/mixed with seltzer water), 2 g net carbs
- Pinot grigio, 3 g net carbs
- Sauvignon blanc, 3 g net carbs
- Chardonnay, 3 g net carbs
- Fumé blanc, 3 g net carbs

- Dry rosé wine, 3 g net carbs

For reference, compare these options to a higher carb white wine, such as:

- White sangria, 8 g net carbs
- White zinfandel, 8 g net carbs

Red Wine Recommendations

- Pinot noir, 3 g net carbs
- Merlot, 4 g net carbs
- Shiraz, 4 g net carbs
- Syrah, 4 g net carbs
- Cabernet sauvignon, 4 g net carbs
- Red zinfandel, 4 g net carbs
- Chianti, 4 g net carbs
- Sangiovese, 4 g net carbs
- Grenache, 4 g net carbs

For reference, compare these options to a higher carb red wine, such as:

- Burgundy, 5 g net carbs
- Red sangria, 12 g net carbs

Because alcohol affects you differently on DIRTY, LAZY, KETO, be responsible and designate a sober driver to get you home safely (with instructions NOT to hit the drive-thru).

DIRTY, LAZY, KETO
FOOD PYRAMID

As a child, do you remember blankly staring at the side of a cereal box while munching on Cap'n Crunch? I can clearly recall wearing my footed pajamas and mindlessly staring at the brightly colored pyramid of USDA guidelines. The tiered approach of DIRTY, LAZY, KETO is reminiscent of this cereal-box graphic, but diverges with its recommendations. Instead of eating the USDA's six to eight servings of grains and cereals, for example, DIRTY, LAZY, KETO emphasizes the value of eating healthy fats, quality protein, and non-starchy vegetables.

There are hundreds of keto pyramid guides on Pinterest, but not one DIRTY, LAZY, KETO pyramid. In fact, I made this one up! (see p. 91.) I even hired a graphic designer to make it pretty for you. If you are familiar with the "real deal" ketogenic diet, where upward of 70 percent of calories derive from fat, you will immediately notice that my pyramid is different. Instead of asking you to eat fat, fat, and more fat, I am recommending you enjoy the majority of calories from not *just* healthy fat, but protein, *and* non-starchy vegetables, too. In fact, I would like to stress that eating those three things will bring you the most success in your weight-loss journey. This was how I lost 140 pounds, in a nutshell! Yes, I did enjoy full-fat dairy, and some nuts, seeds, and fruit, but the majority of what I ate fell into these three big categories: **healthy fats, quality proteins, and non-starchy vegetables.**

An overall theme of the DIRTY, LAZY, KETO food pyramid is to eat fewer net carbohydrates. By keeping your blood sugar stable, you will stop the spike, crash, and overeating cycle that has historically caused you and I so much trouble. There is a method to the madness, people. Even if you disagree with my strategy, the outcome of following DIRTY, LAZY, KETO is stunning. You just can't argue with actual results!

You might get angry or have strong reactions to what's *not* on the DIRTY, LAZY, KETO pyramid. It's totally understandable for you to question my recommendations, since they are *so incredibly different* from what we've been taught *for our entire lives*. Take fruit, for example; you might be thinking to yourself, "How in the world can eating fruit make me fat?" I understand how harebrained this all sounds at first, and I can see how you might feel suspicious. Expecting you to turn your back on USDA guidelines might feel confusing and wrong, like I'm asking you to cheat on taxes.

Either way, I appreciate that you are feeling surprised about what foods are sanctioned by DIRTY, LAZY, KETO. This blueprint for losing weight falls into some kind of nutritious "loophole," for sure, but honestly, *who cares*? Whether "right" or "wrong," all I know is that by eating this way, I

DIRTY, LAZY, KETO FOOD PYRAMID

A visual representation of how 20–50g of net carbs per day could be spent

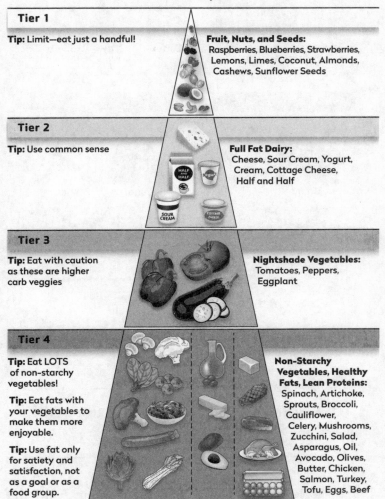

Tier 1

Tip: Limit—eat just a handful!

Fruit, Nuts, and Seeds: Raspberries, Blueberries, Strawberries, Lemons, Limes, Coconut, Almonds, Cashews, Sunflower Seeds

Tier 2

Tip: Use common sense

Full Fat Dairy: Cheese, Sour Cream, Yogurt, Cream, Cottage Cheese, Half and Half

Tier 3

Tip: Eat with caution as these are higher carb veggies

Nightshade Vegetables: Tomatoes, Peppers, Eggplant

Tier 4

Tip: Eat LOTS of non-starchy vegetables!

Tip: Eat fats with your vegetables to make them more enjoyable.

Tip: Use fat only for satiety and satisfaction, not as a goal or as a food group.

Non-Starchy Vegetables, Healthy Fats, Lean Proteins: Spinach, Artichoke, Sprouts, Broccoli, Cauliflower, Celery, Mushrooms, Zucchini, Salad, Asparagus, Oil, Avocado, Olives, Butter, Chicken, Salmon, Turkey, Tofu, Eggs, Beef

Lean protein, non-starchy vegetables, and healthy fats will help keep you full!

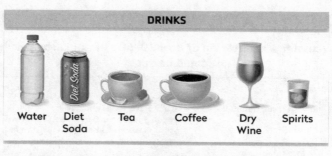

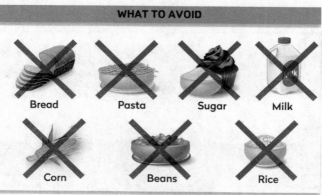

lost half of my entire body weight. I've kept the weight off now for seven years and counting, and *it's not that hard.*

I absolutely know with all of my heart that this will work for you, too.

Let's get over ourselves, stop arguing about fruit, and learn how to figure out the logistics of getting you started, *capisce?*

The pyramid is designed to give you a "visual representation" of what your overall eating in a day might look like. This is not an exact science. You do not have to "check the box" for eating foods from each category. Unlike other keto programs with prepared goals, limits, and ratios, with DIRTY, LAZY, KETO, the net carbs are yours to spend *how you see fit*. That's what makes this program sustainable, in my opinion. That being said, I'd like to give you a broad explanation about what future eating patterns might look like. Do I need to say it again? This is your life. Eat what makes sense to you! With common sense and a personal mission to change your eating habits, use the DIRTY, LAZY, KETO pyramid only as inspiration and guidance while you make independent choices.

TIER 1: JUST A HANDFUL—Fruit

Starting at the top of the pyramid, you will see that DIRTY, LAZY, KETO recommends eating only a small amount of low-carb fruits. This is not because fruits are bad for you; I'm not saying that at all! Fruits are delicious, but unfortunately, also naturally very sweet. Because of the natural sugar they contain, fruits are carbohydrate dense. We have discussed how high-carbohydrate foods can cause blood sugar to spike and crash, which often starts the cycle of eating again to improve one's energy level. For this reason, I recommend eating only low-net-carbs fruits, and in small amounts.

That being said, if you love eating watermelon (remember that story?), you can still eat some freaking watermelon!

This is your life and you need to make DIRTY, LAZY, KETO work for you. Don't quit a "diet" because a food isn't listed as "allowable." There is always another way. DIRTY, LAZY, KETO is a lifestyle—make this work for you!

Make an informed decision about whether you eat that forbidden item, or substitute something with a similar flavor to get your "fix." Not to beat the watermelon example to death or anything, but instead of eating excessive amounts of watermelon, what about having watermelon-infused water? Or would watermelon-flavored, sugar-free gum help? If one of these suggestions doesn't work for you, then eat some watermelon already! *Recognize, however, that what you "love to eat" might have a metabolic effect that causes an undesirable chain reaction.* Even when I eat too much of something "healthy" like fruit, my energy level quickly spikes when the fructose (sugar) in fruit is quickly converted into glucose for immediate energy use. If I don't "burn up" that energy quickly (like with exercise), the excess glucose is stored as fat. Maybe save watermelon and other higher-carb fruits to enjoy on a day where you know you'll be more active. That way, you have an opportunity to "burn off" those carbs, and they won't sabotage your weight-loss efforts. Do I have to keep saying this, or can you agree I'm onto something here?

To help put my theory into practical terms, let me offer a useful suggestion. Think of berries or low-net carb fruits like a "topping" and not a food group. They can be enjoyed, but in small amounts. A few berries on top of yogurt, or a handful within a smoothie might provide all the natural sweetness you need to get through a craving. (The net carb count per cup provided here is for your reference only, not a suggestion for your serving size.) Enjoy a sprinkle or small handful of low-carb fruit and move on with your day.

"Lower-Carb" Recommended Fruits

Avocado, 1 g net carbs per ⅓ of a medium (50 gram) avocado serving

Blackberries, 6 g net carbs per 1 cup serving

Blueberries, 18 g net carbs per 1 cup serving—*Don't eat the whole cup, people!*

Coconut (unsweetened, shredded), 2 g net carbs per 2 tablespoon serving

Lemon (fresh), 4 g net carbs per medium fruit (2⅛" in diameter) serving

Lime (fresh), 5 g net carbs per medium fruit (2⅛" in diameter) serving

Raspberries, 7 g net carbs per 1 cup serving

Rhubarb,* 3 g net carbs per 1 cup serving

Starfruit, 4 g net carbs per 1 cup serving

Strawberries, 8 g net carbs per 1 cup serving

TIER 1: JUST A HANDFUL—Nuts and Seeds

Also, in the "limit" range are nuts and seeds. I could eat these suckers all day long! Nuts and seeds are calorie dense and easy to overeat (common sense!), so these land at the top of

---

* Rhubarb is technically a vegetable, but it's often sweetened and prepared as a fruit in desserts.

the pyramid. Even with the added fiber, it's hard to stop eating these. What follows is not a complete list, but a reference to get you started when deciding which nuts and seeds to eat. Again, note the net carbs are *per ounce* as a uniform reference. I'm just giving you that information to consider. But instead of making yourself stressed out with meticulous measuring, try a "chill" system of enjoying a small handful.

Nuts

Almonds, 3 g net carbs per 1 oz.

Brazil nuts, 1 g net carb per 1 oz. serving

Coconut (unsweetened, shredded), 2 g net carbs per 1 oz. serving

Hazelnuts, 2 g net carbs per 1 oz. serving

Macadamia nuts, 2 g net carbs per 1 oz. serving

Peanuts (roasted, salted), 3 g net carbs per 1 oz. serving

Pecan nuts (halves), 1 g net carbs per 1 oz. serving

Walnut (halves and pieces), 2 g net carbs per 1 oz. serving

Seeds

Chia seeds (black, whole), 3 g net carb per 1 oz. serving

Flaxseed (ground), 1 g net carb per 1 oz. serving

Flaxseed meal (whole), 2 g net carb per 1 oz. serving

Hemp seeds (shelled), 1 g net carbs per 1 oz. serving

Pumpkin seeds (roasted and salted), 2 g net carbs per
   1 oz. serving
Sesame seeds (raw), 4 g net carbs per 1 oz. serving
Sunflower seeds, 4 g net carbs per 1 oz. serving

TIER 2: FULL-FAT DAIRY

Delicious dairy! Yogurt, milk, cheese, and cream—SERIOUSLY!
How can all of this deliciousness be encouraged? *So exciting,* people. If you have any anger about losing your beloved
pasta, please take a moment and thank the dairy category for
making the hit list of DIRTY, LAZY, KETO.

Considering that your daily net carbs spending likely
falls between 20 and 50 grams (depending on your body
type, activity, and what is working best for your lifestyle),
you have to be careful when consuming dairy, as you do
with nuts, seeds, and fruits. Because dairy and these other
foods are so delicious, it is easy to go overboard and "use
up" all of your carb budget at once. These foods are to be
enjoyed, but in moderation. To maintain healthy digestion,
you need to save room in your carb expenditure for fibrous
vegetables.

When searching for dairy foods to enjoy, here are some tips:

Yogurt

High-fat, plain yogurt has the lowest level of carbohydrates
possible. I usually buy whatever is on sale and am still able

to find yogurts in the 2–8 grams net carbs per cup serving range. If the yogurt doesn't have enough fat for my liking, I sprinkle unsweetened shredded coconut or macadamia nuts on top to boost the nutritional content. Some popular brands of keto-friendly yogurt include: Fage Total 5%, TWO GOOD, Chobani, YO by Yoplait, Oikos, and house-branded plain Greek yogurt without added sugar.

Do you have to eat yogurt? Of course you don't; you will be passing up a great source of calcium, however. I frequently eat yogurt with a sprinkle of berries on top. Note that this combination might add up to ten carbs or more—*I'm wild and crazy like that!* Another breakfast favorite of mine is to mix unsweetened cocoa powder and zero-carbs sweetener into my yogurt. This sugar-free concoction reminds me of the chocolate pudding found at a restaurant salad bar. The combinations with yogurt are endless. You can even mix a sugar-free drink flavor packet with yogurt for a fun, fruity flavor. *Who knew?*

Milk

Regular milk, even full-fat or low-fat milk, remains high in carbs due to the lactose component. To substitute, the alternative-milk market has broadened in recent years and is almost negligible in sugar. Yes, dairy-alternative drinks still contain carbs, but not as many as you might expect. Almond milk, cashew milk, hemp milk, and soy milk are examples of lactose-free, unsweetened "dairy" beverages. These beauties are great to have on hand for creamy recipes or even as a smoothie mixer. Be open-minded and give these a try. You might surprise yourself and fall in love with one.

Be sure to check the label of your milk alternative for specifics, but these net carbs estimates can help guide you:

Almond milk (unsweetened), 1 g net carb per cup
Soy milk (plain or original, unsweetened), 1 g net carb
   per cup
Cashew milk (unsweetened), 1 g net carb per cup
Hemp milk (unsweetened), 0 g net carbs per cup

Cream

A little goes a long way when enjoying the rich, velvety texture of cream. I can put just a splash in my coffee or smoothie for added fat and an overall feeling of decadence. Unfortunately, I hear many keto followers go completely overboard with this seductive ingredient. They add excessive amounts of HWC—to both dessert recipes and gourmet coffee drinks—and then wonder why their weight loss has stalled. Employ some common sense, people! The dairy category hovers at the top of the DIRTY, LAZY, KETO pyramid and should be consumed *only in moderation.*

Heavy whipping cream, 0 g net carbs per 1 tablespoon
   serving
Half-and-half, 1 g net carb per 1 tablespoon serving
Sour cream, 1 g net carb per 2 tablespoon serving

Cheese

Most hard cheeses weigh in between 0 and 1 gram net carbs per serving. Interestingly, the shredded cheeses sold in convenient pouches have more carbs than in the same type of cheese sold in blocks. Manufacturers add potato starch and cellulose fiber to keep the shredded cheese from clumping, which adds to the carb count per serving. Personally, I don't let things like this stop me: I still buy the packaged shredded cheese because of the convenience. This *is* DIRTY, LAZY, KETO, after all! I have learned that the carb count varies among shredded-cheese brands, so I make sure to compare packages before making a purchase. Lastly, note that cheese as a category is decadent and easy to overconsume. Even though the carb count of cheese is at the lower end, I recommend enjoying small amounts. My suggestion is to sprinkle cheese all over your vegetables and protein, rather than to eat cheese as a separate snack. This strategy will help you "slow your roll" when enjoying cheese and will also make your vegetables taste better!

American cheese (processed), 1 g net carb per 1 slice serving

Asiago cheese, 0 g net carb per 1 oz. serving

Blue cheese, 1 g net carb per 1 oz. serving

Brie cheese, 0 g net carb per 1 oz. serving

Cheddar cheese, 1 g net carb per 1 oz. serving

Colby jack cheese, 1 g net carb per 1 oz. serving

Cottage cheese, 4% milk fat, 5 g net carbs per ½ cup serving

Cream cheese, 2–3 g net carbs per 2 tablespoon serving

Feta cheese, 1 g net carb per oz. serving

Gorgonzola cheese, 1 g net carb per 1 oz. serving

Goat cheese, 0 g net carb per 1 oz. serving

Gouda cheese, 0 g net carb per 1 oz. serving

Gruyere cheese, 0 g net carb per 1 oz. serving

Monterey jack cheese, 0 g net carb per 1 oz. serving

Mozzarella cheese, 1 g net carb per 1 oz. serving

Muenster cheese, 0 g net carb per 1 oz. serving

Parmesan cheese, 1 g net carb per 1 oz. serving

Pepper jack cheese, 0 g net carb per 1 oz. serving

Provolone cheese, 1 g net carb per 1 oz. serving

Ricotta cheese (whole milk), 3 g net carb per ¼ cup
serving

String cheese, 1 g net carb per 1 piece (28 gram)
serving

Swiss cheese, 0–1 g net carb per 1 oz. serving

Velveeta cheese, 3 g net carb per 1 oz. serving

TIER 3: ARE ALL VEGETABLES GOOD FOR YOU?

Aren't all vegetables good for you? Not all vegetables are created equal. Some definitely have more carbs than others.

**Thank you, Mr. French Fry, for ruining
the reputation of your entire food group.**

Nightshade vegetables grow in the shade but flower at night. I'm not sure why this is important, but it helps me remember that nightshade vegetables start off as little pranksters. As a category, I learned they have more carbs than other, more innocent vegetables. Examples of nightshade vegetables are eggplant, bell peppers, tomatoes, tomatillos, cayenne peppers, and potatoes. Potatoes, however, offer the greatest number of carbs in the nightshade category. I *do not* consider potatoes, *even sweet potatoes,* to be keto-friendly. Be aware of the higher level of carbohydrates of the entire nightshade category when planning meals, recipes, and snacks. For example, I put thin slices of tomato on my salad, but I don't eat an entire plate of tomatoes with basil. See the difference?

On a side note, some folks have negative physical reactions to eating nightshade vegetables. Reactions include diarrhea, bloating, headaches, gas, or even pain in the joints.

Nightshade Vegetables

Tomatillo, 1 g net carb per ¼ cup serving

Tomatoes, 5 g net carbs per 1 cup serving

Green bell peppers, 4 g net carbs per 1 cup serving

Yellow bell peppers, 8 g net carbs per 1 cup serving

Red bell peppers, 12 g net carbs per 1 cup serving

Jalapeño peppers, 3 g net carbs per 1 cup serving

Eggplant, 2 g net carbs per 1 cup serving

Beyond the nightshade category, vegetables still vary in terms of carb count. Some argue the rule that "aboveground" vegetables have fewer carbs than "belowground" vegetables, but even so, there are exceptions. My recommendation is to look up the nutritional value for what you are eating, then plan accordingly.

Quick tip: Did you know you can "ask Siri," "ask Google," or (my favorite) "ask Alexa" for a carb count on a food? I find this more convenient than using an app. Plus, I can never seem to find my phone.

TIER 4: NON-STARCHY VEGETABLES

What can I binge eat? Surprise—non-starchy vegetables! *(I bet that was definitely NOT the answer you were hoping to hear!)*

The coffers finally start to open with the category of non-starchy vegetables. FINALLY! Eat up, sister (or brother!). Eat to your heart's content. If you're like me, you might NOT have a built in "off switch" when it comes to eating. I need to eat in bulk, so this is my favorite category. Find recipes that work with your lifestyle and family's needs, and incorporate large amounts of non-starchy vegetables into your regimen. Ideally, you want to consume these at every stinkin' meal. If it helps you swallow this information (*get it, swallow?*), you can coat these suckers in the fat of your choice to make them more tolerable. I hope I haven't lost you on this one. (Stay tuned, steak is coming!) I'm going to give this category a lot

of airtime, as I can't say enough about the weight-loss prop-
erties of these veggies.

Non-starchy Recommended Vegetables

Alfalfa sprouts, 0 g net carbs per 1 cup serving

Artichoke, 5 g net carbs per ½ cup serving

Arugula, 1 g net carb per 1 cup serving

Asparagus, 2 g net carbs per 1 cup serving

Bamboo shoots, 5 g net carbs per 1 cup

Bean sprouts, 4 g net carbs per 1 cup serving

Beans (green, wax, Italian), 2 g net carbs per ½ cup
    serving

Bell pepper (green), 4 g net carbs per 1 cup serving

Bell pepper (red), 12 g net carbs per 1 cup serving

Bell pepper (yellow), 8 g net carbs per 1 cup serving

Broccoli (fresh), 4 g net carbs per 1 cup serving

Broccoli (frozen), 2 g net carbs per 1 cup serving

Brussels sprouts (cooked from fresh), 3 g net carbs
    per ½ cup serving

Cabbage (bok choy), 1 g net carb per 1 cup serving

Cabbage (green, raw), 3 g net carbs per 1½ cup serving

Cauliflower (raw), 3 g net carbs per 1 cup serving

Cauliflower (riced), 2 g net carbs per ½ cup serving

Celery (raw), 1 g net carb per 1 cup serving

Chayote, 4 g net carbs per 1 cup serving

Chicory greens, 0 g net carbs per 1 cup serving

Chinese cabbage, 1 g net carb per 1 cup serving

Cole slaw mix, 3 g net carbs per 1½ cup serving

Collard greens (cooked), 3 g net carbs per 1 cup serving

Cucumber (raw), 2 g net carbs per 1 cup serving

Daikon (oriental radish, raw), 3 g net carbs per 1 cup serving

Edamame, 4 g net carbs per ½ cup serving

Eggplant, 2 g net carbs per 1 cup serving

Endive, 0 g net carb per 1 cup serving

Escarole, 1 g net carb per 1 cup serving

Green bean (string, raw), 4 g net carbs per 1 cup serving

Green onion (raw), 4 g net carb per 1 cup serving

Greens (collard, cooked), 3 g net carbs per 1 cup serving

Greens (kale, cooked from fresh), 2 g net carbs per ½ cup serving

Heart of palm (canned), 3 g net carb per 1 cup serving

Jalapeño (fresh), 1 g net carb per ¼ cup serving

Kale (cooked), 2 g net carbs per ½ cup serving

Leeks (cooked), 6 g net carbs per ½ cup serving

Lettuce and salad mixes, 1–2 g net carbs per 2 cup serving

Mushroom (raw), 2 g net carb per 1 cup serving

Mustard greens, 1 g net carb per 1 cup serving

Okra, 4 g net carb per 1 cup serving

Onion (red, yellow, white), 12 g net carbs per 1 cup serving

Snow peas, 4 g net carbs per 1½ cup serving

Peperoncini (sliced), 0–1 g net carbs per 12 piece (30 gram) serving

Radicchio lettuce, 1 g net carb per 1 cup serving

Radish, 2 g net carbs per 1 cup serving

Red onion, 12 g net carbs per 1 cup serving

Rhubarb, 3 g net carbs per 1 cup serving
Romaine lettuce, 1 g net carb per 1 cup serving
Rutabaga (raw), 9 g net carbs per 1 cup serving
Salad greens, 0–1 g net carbs per 2 cups serving
Snap pea, 4 g net carbs per 1½ cup serving
Spinach (raw), 0 g net carb per 1 cup serving
Sprout (alfalfa), 0 g net carbs per 1 cup serving
Swiss chard, 2 g net carbs per ½ cup serving
Tomatillo, 1 g net carb per ¼ cup serving
Tomato, 4 g net carbs per 1 medium-sized whole fruit
    (123 gram) serving
White onion, 12 g net carbs per 1 cup serving
Yellow onion, 12 g net carbs per cup serving
Zucchini, 3 g net carbs per 1 cup (chopped) serving
Zucchini, 2 g net carbs per 1 cup (sliced) serving

TIER 4: PROTEIN

When I first started eating DIRTY, LAZY, KETO, something that surprised me was how aware I became about the lack of protein I had previously been eating. When I changed that eating pattern and began eating protein at every meal, there was an immediate positive effect. I felt more satisfied after finishing the meal, I ate less overall, and I wasn't hungry again for a while. WEIRD! My armchair analysis is that previously I was stuck in a carbohydrate-addicted cycle of false energy. I had no idea what sustainable energy even felt like. WOW! Let me tell you, it's a huge change for the better.

I know lots of "keto experts" warn against eating too much protein. They tout concerns about how excessive protein calories turning into carbs, or something metabolically complicated like that. I'm sure all of this is true, but I don't think this reasoning explains why I was overweight most of my adult life. It surely wasn't from overeating eggs, chicken, or fish, *no, ma'am*. Let's be real here! Have you heard the joke "Don't blame the butter for what the bread did?" Well I'd like to expand that joke to include "Don't blame the protein for what the carbs did." *(Okay, that wasn't very funny; whatever!)* You get my point, right? Unless you are dumping protein powder on everything you are eating, I doubt excessive chicken eating is to blame for your historic weight problem.

There are a wide range of proteins available to meet your budgets and tastes. I encourage you to eat "real protein" whenever possible and enjoy processed meat in moderation. Hot dogs and jerky, aka "keto junk food," are allowed with DIRTY, LAZY, KETO (*yeah!*) but shouldn't represent the bulk of your choices. *Do the best you can.* Use common sense here to enjoy a variety of high-quality proteins. (Notice I didn't say "expensive.") Some strategies to save on groceries include being flexible to eat what's on sale, buying in bulk, and freezing meats.

DIRTY, LAZY, KETO Protein Ideas

Bacon (unflavored), 0 g net carbs per 2 cooked slices
    (19 gram)
Beef, 0 g net carbs per 3 oz. serving

Chicken, 0 g net carbs per 4 oz. serving

Duck, 0 g net carbs per 4 oz. serving

Eggs, 1 g net carbs per medium egg serving

Fish and shellfish, 0 g net carbs per 3 oz. serving

Gyro meat, 5–7 g net carbs per 2 oz. serving

Hot dogs, varies per brand, estimated 2 g net carbs
    per 1 link (42 g) serving

Jerky, varies per brand, estimated 3 g net carbs per
    serving

Lamb, 0 g net carbs per serving

Lunch meat, varies per brand, estimated 0–2 g net carbs
    per 2 oz serving

Pepperoni, 0 g net carbs per 15 slice (28 gram) serving

Pork, 0 g net carbs per 3 oz. serving

Tofu, 1–2 g net carbs per 3 oz. (1″ slice) serving

Turkey, 0 g net carbs per 3 oz. serving

TVP (textured vegetable protein meat substitute), 1–15 g
    net carb per serving, as this varies per protein style
    (nuggets, crumbles, burgers, etc.)

TIER 4: HEALTHY FATS AND OILS

Fat is fabulous. Fat helps everything you eat literally slide through your digestive system and out the other end! **Fat is satiating and makes you feel, well, *like you're not on a diet.*** Not feeling deprived has been critical to my success. I suspect fats are the key to why I have been able to stick with DIRTY, LAZY, KETO for seven years now. I've realized this isn't a diet, it's a lifestyle. Actually, I feel pretty scandalous when I order a salad at lunch covered in blue cheese dressing, with an extra side of dressing! I love ordering like that, especially when I'm sitting in a restaurant with "hangry" dieters picking at their plain lettuce. **I don't feel resentful when I eat. I actually feel content. This feeling is important for long-term success!**

As a macronutrient category, I'm quite aware that there are "good fats" and "bad fats." In my own weight-loss journey, I didn't discern between monosaturated fats, polyunsaturated fats, or omega-3 fatty acids. I just used common sense and ate within my family's limited budget. I didn't buy Kerrygold brand butter (considered to be the "gold standard" of keto dieters); in fact, as of yet I haven't even tried it. I shop at Walmart and other discount retailers for my groceries. I use all sorts of cooking oils, cheap mayonnaise (gasp!), generic dairy products, nuts from vending machines, and dollar-store salad dressings as my fat sources. That being said, I do encourage you to eat the healthiest fats available! This is an example of "Do as I say, not as I do." I aim to improve myself in this category.

Eating excessive grams of fat is not a goal of DIRTY, LAZY, KETO.

#BreakTheRules

There is no fat minimum or gram counting here, just a sprinkling of common sense. You are not "required" to eat a certain amount of fat. I never did! I made sure to *incorporate fats into every meal,* but I *did not* make meals out of fat alone. For example, I cook meats using oil. I top my salads with creamy salad dressing. I serve vegetables with melted butter. I DON'T EAT SPOONFULS OF COCONUT OIL OR CUBES OF BUTTER at the end of the night to "get my fats in." This is an important distinction between DIRTY, LAZY, KETO and the traditional strict keto diet you may have read about.

Since we are on the topic of fat, I can't continue without talking about the infamous FAT BOMB. Somebody pull out a soapbox, because I need somewhere to stand. When I hear about people eating "fat bombs" to meet a fat goal, I cringe. Instead of making fat bomb desserts, I use fats to make healthy eating more tolerable. Sautéing vegetables with fat (rather than eating fat for fat's sake) or dipping artichoke leaves in mayo are specific examples of what I'm talking about here.

You might be worried about DIRTY, LAZY, KETO and your cholesterol levels at this point. Again, I direct you to work with your health-care provider for specific guidance. I can only attest to my own personal experience when responding to this topic. Before starting DIRTY, LAZY, KETO, weighing upward of 300 pounds, my cholesterol levels were also north of 300. That's not surprising at all, right? What did floor me, however, was how dramatically my cholesterol levels dropped after losing weight while eating so much fat on DIRTY, LAZY, KETO. WEIRD! Since a cholesterol test is a measure of how much fat is in your blood, why did my levels drop to "normal range"? I honestly have no idea! My doctor was also blown away. My unscientific opinion is that the fibrous vegetables I eat, lubed by healthy fats, scrub away the crusty plaque that was built up my arteries from years of overeating Cap'n Crunch.

Not everyone will experience normal cholesterol levels on a keto diet. Your body is unique! Partnering with your doctor is key here. Cholesterol is just one marker of your overall heart health, and you must monitor all of your risk factors with a trained professional. I asked Dr. Mike Jones (the obesity specialist who wrote the foreword for this book) to weigh in about this topic from a medical perspective:

"In those using a ketogenic diet as part of the treatment of obesity, I would suggest that even if it were shown to pose some increased risk, the benefit of a significant and sustained reduction in body fat mass will almost always outweigh such risk." *

DIRTY, LAZY, KETO Fat and Oil Ideas

Avocado, 1 g net carbs per ⅓ of a medium (50 gram) avocado serving

Brazil nuts, 1 g net carb per 1 oz. serving

Butter, 0 g net carbs per 1 tablespoon serving

Cheese, 0–1 g net carbs per 1 oz. serving

Coconut (unsweetened, shredded), 2 g net carbs per 2 tablespoon serving

Coconut milk (unsweetened, 12–14% fat), 1 g net carbs per 2.7 fl. oz. or ⅓ cup serving

---

* https://www.ncbi.nlm.nih.gov/pmc/articles/PMC2716748

Cottage cheese, 4% milkfat, 5 g net carbs per ½ cup
serving

Cream cheese, 2–3 g net carbs per 2 tablespoon
serving

Ghee, 0 g net carbs per 1 tablespoon serving

Half-and-half (full-fat), 1 g net carb per 2 tablespoon
serving

Hazelnuts, 2 g net carbs per 1 oz. serving

Heavy whipping cream, 0 g net carbs per 1 tablespoon
serving

Macadamia nuts, 2 g net carbs per 1 oz. serving

Mayonnaise (full-fat), 0 g net carbs per 1 tablespoon
serving

MCT oil, 0 g net carbs per 1 tablespoon serving*

Oil (canola, coconut, grapeseed, olive, peanut, sesame,
sunflower, safflower, walnut), 0 g net carb per
1 tablespoon serving

Olives (black, green), 1 g net carb per 2 (large)
olive serving, 1 g net carb per 5 (medium) olive
serving

Pecan nuts (halves), 1 g net carbs per ¼ cup
serving

Salad dressing, varies depending on brand, estimated
1–3 g net carbs per 2 tablespoon serving

Salmon, 0 g net carbs per 3 oz. serving

Sour cream, 1 g net carbs per 2 tablespoon serving

Yogurt, varies depending on brand, estimated 3–9 g
net carbs per cup serving

---

* I don't use MCT oil, personally, but if I don't mention it, I'm sure to get complaints!

Is That All You Need? *Not So Fast*

Understanding the DIRTY, LAZY, KETO pyramid isn't enough. I don't know about you, but I visit my kitchen dozens of times a day *when I'm not even hungry.* What am I looking for inside my fridge?

**Food won't solve my problems, but
I keep looking there for answers.**

By repeatedly opening pantry doors, it seems I am hoping a magic portal will appear. Do I hope to be surprised with something other than food on the inside of the cabinet? I wonder sometimes what it is I am looking for by wandering into the kitchen so often. Instead of a snack, do I desire something more? Maybe I'm yearning for a friend because I feel lonely, or for comfort because I feel stressed. Instead of a sandwich, what is it that I really want?

What do I really need that I keep looking for with food?

Changing *what* we eat is simple, but changing *why* we eat is an entirely different matter. I want to help you explore both sides of this complicated issue. I want you to lose weight, yes, but even more critical, I want you to help yourself figure out *how to keep that weight off.* Our problems run deeper than just what's stocked inside our cupboards and fridge. It's naïve to think cutting carbs alone will solve our problems. If we don't address the whole picture, obesity will come back like a bad rash.

Now I'm not a therapist, you know that, but I am a woman who, against all the odds, *somehow figured this shit out.* Let me help guide you through the rest of your weight-loss journey. Together, we will address precisely how to make DIRTY, LAZY, KETO into a comprehensive lifestyle.

Without any further *adieu,* let's get crackin'!

1

WHY AREN'T WE THIN ALREADY?

Why You Failed in the Past

I'm addicted to reality television shows about weight loss. I love to root for underdogs, as I see myself in their same shoes. No matter what age or background the contestants come from, I see similarities between their challenges and my own struggles. My only bone to pick with these shows is the mock, off-camera interviews. Inevitably, a producer uncovers the *single tragic event* responsible for a contestant's obesity in just a few minutes. *As if finding the cause for being overweight were that simple.*

In my own experience, there was never "just one thing" that led me to become severely overweight.

The most obvious reason for my obesity was that I really liked eating—and still do! The sad truth is that I ate too much of the wrong things. While it might seem obvious, I'll admit the truth—I didn't know "how to eat right." My husband thinks that's funny.

"Of course, you know how to eat right," he pokes; "that's ridiculous." (Mind you, he is quite thin.)

"Just eat healthy foods!" he exclaims, thinking the problem is solved. I think weight loss is a lot more complicated than that, and I suspect you just might agree.

When people ask me, "What made you finally decide to lose the weight?" I've been known to sarcastically reply, "Well, I really liked being fat!"

I give a dumb answer to an even dumber question. No one wants to be overweight or obese. No one wants to be stared at, or worse, be ignored. I spent years fearing the dressing room because I knew the clothes wouldn't fit. I avoided restaurants with booths because I couldn't sit comfortably between the seat and the table. I sweated constantly. I awkwardly stood at social events rather than risk an embarrassing collapse of a provided flimsy plastic chair under my extra weight. I pretended not to want to go on amusement park rides, knowing I might not fit in the car. I felt uncomfortable *just being alive*.

People who have never struggled with their weight *don't really get it*. They sometimes think weight-loss surgery must be the answer for people like me. Now, I didn't have surgery, though I admit it crossed my mind. But when one of my coworkers chose to have the lap-band, I became curious to learn more. I had known a few people who had completed the gastric bypass surgery, but this new procedure was becoming more popular. Could the lap-band be a cure for obesity? As much as I loved living in denial, hearing about my friend's elective surgery made me stop and think about my options. I came home from work that night and checked my health insurance website to see if the lap-band was a covered benefit. After researching online, I discovered my BMI of 45 percent qualified me for insurance coverage. The fact that I was even considering surgery made me terribly sad. I didn't want to do anything about my weight. *I just wanted to ignore it.* But with a BMI showing me that almost HALF of my body was ALL fat? Well, I felt I had to *do* something. *But what?*

I was stunned by my situation. I saw myself as such a determined, capable person who had always been able to succeed no matter how challenging my goals. I finished college at the top of my class while juggling multiple jobs and even went on to complete graduate school. How could I be so successful in one part of my life but an utter failure at the rest? It didn't make any sense.

Why couldn't I lose weight on my own? I felt hopeless and alone. It seemed no matter what diet I tried, nothing worked.

With a success rate of 1 percent, diets across the board apparently don't work for anyone. Wow, that's gloomy. It's a wonder people even try! Imagine if a doctor prescribed an expensive medication for you but added the caveat, "Oh, this might work only for a little while. Actually, it cures the underlying problem about one percent of the time."

Would you still take the medicine? I probably wouldn't. That sounds like a waste of my time and money. What about you? Would you try that medicine with a miserable 1 percent success rate?

I find this topic absolutely fascinating. Diets, in all their shapes and sizes, all have the same goal: they aim to help you reach that 1 percent success rate. We are all so desperate for a cure that we are willing to try anything. I know I've tried every diet on the planet with varying results. Who hasn't? Eat soup all day? CHECK! Replace my meals with shakes? CHECK! As a nation, we are willing to do just about anything to become part of the 1 percent. We are desperate for any solution, even willing to try those diets that have outlandish sacrifices.

As the years tick by, though, Facebook reminds me I am still part of the 1 percent. Don't you just love those look-back photos? For me, when I see photos from years ago on social media, the first thing that goes through my mind is, "What size was I there?" *Super obnoxious, I know.* Like a carnival barker, I can accurately tell you my weight within a few pounds *in any photo* you put in front of me. When I see a photo from when I was heavy, I feel so sad. The pictures where I weighed less, though? Those make me feel so proud of my accomplishment. I never want to regain that weight! In order for that to happen, I have analyzed what personal changes I made that supported my weight loss. I need to remind myself *how* I got to this point to prevent any potential backsliding.

I'm on my seventh year maintaining my weight loss, so I've had plenty of time to gather insight.

**My message will be controversial, but
I'm going to speak the damn truth!**

Before I can dispense any weight-loss advice, I need to make sure you're up for the hard work in front of you. I don't want you quitting for any reason, so let's start by addressing the common reasons most people have failed in the past. Do any of these reasons resonate with you?

I Quit! Common Reasons People Stop a Diet

Deprivation

"I'm hangry."

Calorie deprivation leads to hunger.

Resentment

"But everyone else is having some."

"This isn't fair."

Dieters quit when they feel they are missing out.

All or Nothing

"I slipped up. Forget the whole thing!"

People think they have to follow a diet perfectly or not at all.

Too Expensive

"I can't afford this."

Dieters convince themselves that losing weight requires costly ingredients, meal plans, and exclusive memberships.

Denial

"I'm fine just the way I am."

People quit diets after convincing themselves their weight isn't a problem.

No Support

"My family won't eat this weird food."

With no one on their side, people quit diets when they feel alone.

Cheating

"I'm such a failure."

After one "bad" choice, people feel terrible about themselves and enter a guilt/shame/eating cycle.

Impatience

"I only lost ten pounds this month."

It's not working fast enough.

Self-Esteem

"I'm not attractive at any weight."

Insecurity makes a person give up before even starting.

Unrealistic Goals

"I should be able to have that."

"I want to fit in my wedding dress."

They want it all.

Temporary Fix

"I can only do this for two weeks."

Dieters quit after achieving a short-term goal, like losing weight for an upcoming cruise.

Don't Really Want to Succeed

"I feel uncomfortable when people notice my figure."

Losing weight changes your appearance and can make you feel vulnerable.

Hopefully you've identified with *at least one* of these reasons for quitting a diet. Why would I say such a thing? If you used one of these excuses in the past, you are likely to use it again. Most of us will revert to the same excuses over and over.

You must uncover the reasons why you have failed at diets in the past or you'll never be able to move forward.

By taking an honest inventory of your past reasons for giving up, you will be able to identify that same excuse if it should pop up again (because the chances are high!). You will be ready to identify the excuse before it can cause trouble. Before we get started with DIRTY, LAZY, KETO, you must anticipate potential obstacles in your way.

Lies and myths keep us from weight-loss success. Some of these fabrications are more complex than others, but they all require attention. How did I come up with this list, you might wonder? Let me tell you: *This was my list*! I told myself every single one of these lies for a really long time. I had to chip away at these hurdles and blindly trust the DIRTY, LAZY, KETO journey, even though it was pitch-dark at times. No one came to rescue me. No one fixed my problems. I had to do it all myself. Though painful to admit, I finally learned that **I had to be the one to change if I wanted a different outcome.**

Expect progress, not perfection, from yourself. There is something unexpectedly beautiful waiting for you on the other side. Ready?

"As long as you are walking, you are on the right path." —Buddhist saying

---

2

I ONLY LOST TEN POUNDS THIS MONTH!

Create Realistic, Personalized Goals

Gymnastics and the Scale

Getting on the scale after a hiatus really sucks. There is no other way to say it. Even today, 140 pounds lighter, I balance myself like a gymnast on the bathroom scale, hoping that standing on one leg will subtract a few pounds. To manipulate how much I weigh, I'll use the bathroom (*multiple times*), take off every bit of jewelry, and even strip down bare naked. (Don't act like you don't do these things!) The scale is powerful. *Seeing* how much we weigh evokes such an emotional response inside that it's almost scary.

There's no way around it, though. In order to get started, we have to know where you've been.

Your life is happening right now. You can't waste another minute in denial. Get on the scale, already!

Yes, stepping on the scale is alarming, especially when you haven't been on it in a while. Believe me, I've been there! I spent years, YEARS, having no clue what my weight was. I even avoided going to the doctor to sidestep facing reality. I could suffer a bout of pneumonia and still not go to the clinic. *I understand.*

Instead of waiting for the ubiquitous "Monday," I want you to do just one thing today: find out how much you weigh. The best things in life are often scary. Today, you'll need to be brave. If you need a little pep talk, here it goes: *choose the bigger life.* Don't let the second half of your life be a shadow of the first. None of this weight-loss business is going to happen until you begin doing it. *Today is the day!* Learning your actual weight is the first step toward a new life.

In addition to learning your current weight, I want you to take a picture of yourself. You don't need to dress up in anything fancy or even put makeup on if you don't want to. The photo needs to be of your entire body, not just a headshot. Use a mirror or the timer function on your phone if you are too embarrassed to ask a friend to help. Why are we doing this you might ask? It turns out that a photo of how you actually look *today* really matters. You need to take a good look at yourself. How we *think* of ourselves and what we *actually look like* are often quite different. We need physical evidence of the truth.

I have only a handful of "before" photos myself. Despite being the family photographer, I always hid from the camera. There are entire vacations and holidays from my past when, according to my photo album, *I didn't exist.* If I *was* in the picture, I was sure to hide my oversized figure by using a small child, a stroller, virtually ANYTHING to block my body from the camera. If I was photographed solo, the shot is only from the shoulders on up. Am I alone with these avoidance strategies? I bet scrapbooking moms across the world can relate to having an "edited" family history.

There will be a day when this prescribed "before" photo will be the most treasured photo of your life, so do not skip this step!

Now that you know where you've been, you are able to decide where you're going next. **It's time to set a goal.** This is something that you, and only you, get to decide.

As a veteran of Weight Watchers, I hated being assigned a goal weight. It made no sense to me that a registration pamphlet would authoritatively make such an important and

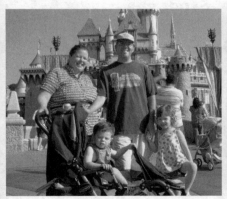 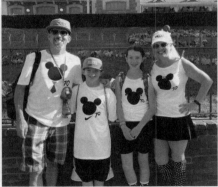

personal decision on my behalf. As a rebel, being told my goal weight probably caused me more harm than good. For my entire life, people have told me what I'm *supposed* to weigh. Why didn't I get a say in this?

#BreakTheRules

Your weight-loss goal doesn't need anyone else's stamp of approval. The goal doesn't even need to align with the evil BMI chart. This is your life and your body; only you get to make decisions about how much you'd like to weigh. Your goal might not even be weight related. For example, your objective might be to lower your blood pressure or to stop taking diabetes medication (under the supervision of your doctor, of course). Maybe you dream of running a 5K race, wearing a ring that hasn't fit in years, or being able to cross your legs with ease. These are acceptable goals! Whatever you chose, write it down. You will be referring back to your goal statement on a regular basis.

"Budda Usta" Syndrome

Empower yourself to choose a weight-loss goal that makes sense only for you, but with one caveat: **you must look forward in time, NOT backward, when choosing your targeted objective.** When you burden yourself with trying to become something or someone you were in the past, my ears perk up like a guard dog alerted to an intruder. I call this dangerous stroll down memory lane the "Budda Usta" syndrome:

- "But I used to . . . weigh 125 in high school."
- "But I used to . . . wear size 6."
- "But I used to . . . go jogging."
- "But I used to . . . be tiny."

Starting a sentence with "But I used to" is a red flag to me. Nostalgia about your past, smaller self undoubtedly drums up feelings of guilt, shame, and anger, none of which are going to help you get started today. Stop living in the past. Obsessing over what happened in high school or what size you wore at your wedding isn't motivating—it's demoralizing. *Let it go already!*

The idea here is to set yourself up for success. **Choose a brand-new goal.** Think about what this goal will look like. Focus brings clarity. By fine-tuning your ambition, you are much more likely to achieve it. I learned this from my mentor, Gretchen Rubin, who asked, "How often do you hit a target when you're not aiming at it?"

All decisions made from this point on will support your path to successful weight loss. If you claim that returning to your high school weight is your goal, think again. Get your head out of the clouds. You're not sixteen anymore! Think about a specific, measurable, achievable, but, most important, *realistic* goal that will actually motivate you.

Be realistic when choosing a goal. See how it stacks up against my criteria:

- Is your goal realistic?
- Is your goal specific?
- Is your goal sustainable?
- Is your goal motivating?
- Is your goal healthy?

Before you begin, I urge you to check in with your physician. Yes, I hate going to the doctor, too. The thought of some perky medical assistant getting all irritated because I want to take an extra minute before stepping on the scale to remove my shoes and set down my purse is enough to raise my blood pressure AT LEAST ten points. If we are being honest here, I would prefer to strip down absolutely naked in order to get the lowest reading possible on that scale *(which might not go over well with the other patients)*.

Checking in with your doctor is needed on many levels. You need to **get a "baseline"** of your current weight, blood pressure, cholesterol, A1C levels, etc. These numbers might feel like a painful reality slap across your face today, but they will be helpful later on. After losing your weight, you will be able to brag about how these stats improved! Imagine how fun it will be to yell, "I TOLD YOU SO!" with *pah-roof* to your keto skeptics. (I LOVE proving people wrong, don't you?)

When I was even moderately overweight, I always felt the doctors "blamed my obesity" for every health problem I sought help for. Whether this was actually substantiated or not, my avoidance of going to the doctor persisted until my weight ballooned to an unprecedented, all-time high close to three hundred pounds. My avoidance was a hurdle I needed to overcome so I could team up with my health-care provider to monitor my new DIRTY, LAZY, KETO lifestyle.

Team up with your family physician when following DIRTY, LAZY, KETO. I'm not a doctor, so I can't verify that this way of eating is appropriate for your current health situation. Your health-care provider can be a source of support and a sounding board. Think of your doctor as your personal consultant. Find a doctor that is educated about the merits of how you plan to lose weight. They are working for you as a paid consultant from your insurance (or pocketbook), so include them as a resource in this process. Be sure to explain what you are eating. You might even bring in this book to share. Be prepared that your doctor might hear "keto" and think you are eating only bacon and butter. That's just not true! Once you educate your doctor about all the vegetables you plan on eating, you will shatter all skepticism.

While your naked butt is sitting on the white paper covering the exam table, take a minute to really drill down to what you are trying to accomplish. You want to develop an emotional connection to your goal. This will become more meaningful than just a clinical number. Imagine what it will feel like and how it will look. Visualize achieving your goal.

I had many goals starting out. Most seemed like faraway dreams at the time, but I want to share my dream with you in the interest of transparency. Here it goes! **I wanted to weigh less than my husband.** It's hard to feel good about yourself when your shirt size is triple that of your beau.

I dreamed of being able to sit on my husband's lap without crushing his entire spirit.

I didn't feel feminine weighing so much more than my husband; it was as simple as that. We travel a lot together, and I wanted to walk onto an airplane and be confident that

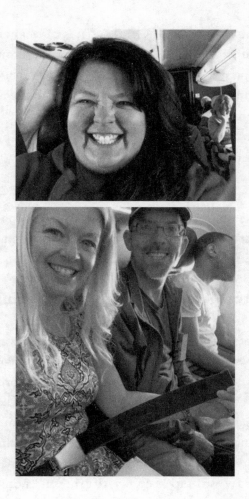

the seat belt would close. When going out to eat, I hoped to sit at a booth, not just a table, without worrying if I could fit in the allotted space. At the movie theater, I didn't want my thighs spilling under the armrest onto my man's chair. Interestingly, my aims changed as I neared the "finish line." Because members of my entire household transitioned their eating habits to mostly DIRTY, LAZY, KETO, my husband's weight became a moving target. Without even trying, he shed thirty-five pounds! *So not fair.* The point is, even with your goal in mind, be open to the fact that goals often evolve during the process.

Oh man, I think I could go on and on here, but I think you get the point.

It's not just a number on the scale I sought after—I wanted a life without embarrassment!

Stop Your Lyin'—Be Accountable

I would not have been able to achieve my goal weight without an honest system to track my progress. We manage what we monitor, and establishing methods early on provided me with motivation and accountability. While you'll have to figure out what kind of system works best for you, I'll share what I found to be helpful. *Of course, I had to learn my lesson the hard way.* After making many mistakes, I finally figured out some easy ways to keep myself truthful, motivated, and on track.

I started changing my eating habits in secret and without a plan, really. The last thing I needed was a bunch of food police circling over my plate espousing unsolicited advice! Starting in secrecy, without a formal announcement to "the world" worked well for me. I was cutting carbs for a good two months before anyone noticed that I was eating differently. This was *in my own house*! In hindsight, I see how the anonymity was a good thing. Having some privacy, especially in the beginning, helped me get my act together and gain keto-confidence. I needed to prove DIRTY, LAZY, KETO worked *to myself* before I could defend it to others.

#BreakTheRules

The way I gained confidence in DIRTY, LAZY, KETO was by actually seeing my weight decrease on my bathroom scale. Like you, I've heard people advise to NEVER get on the scale. "Take measurements instead!" these know-it-alls recommend. *Um, I don't think so.* Not for me, anyway. Measurements might provide *additional information*, but in my opinion, there is no honest substitute for the cold, hard facts provided by the scale. For one, the scale doesn't lie. There is no wiggle room. If I was to rely solely on measurements in lieu of tracking my weight, you can be damn sure that I'd manipulate the system for my benefit. I would suck in my gut, tighten up the tape, and then drive myself to Starbucks to self-sabotage and celebrate the fictitious loss.

The same can be said for using your favorite pants as a so-called measuring stick. If I relied primarily on how my clothes were fitting for feedback about my weight, I would live in leggings or just buy new pants. My weight could go up two sizes before I'd admit to falling off the wagon. Monitoring how clothes fit wouldn't give me an accurate barometer of how I was actually doing.

I'm convinced the scale is the only honest option. Every morning and every night, I religiously hop on the scale. *Yup, I'm that obsessive.* I went from not getting on a scale *for years* to a twice-daily regimen. Instead of using pee strips to see if I'm in ketosis (which I don't recommend, by the way), my scale provides 100 percent accurate feedback. I keep track of my weight in the notes section of my iPhone. With so many entries, I have enough data to predict what will happen in the future. Looking at my weight logged into my phone after the fact doesn't feel as intimidating as seeing the number live on the scale. By removing emotion from the data, I can objectively monitor weight fluctuations. I'm sure there is an app to do all of this, but I like this old-school method.

I became curious to understand why my weight would go up and down at the same time each month. Sure, salty foods, constipation, or overeating had an effect on my weight. But there was a bigger issue at play that I had never considered: *hormones*. Understanding the impact hormones had on my weight was critical to not becoming frustrated with trying to lose weight (and potentially giving up). Right before my period, my weight crept up a bit (causing PANIC, I'll admit), but then afterward, these same pounds would immediately fall off (*relief!*). Getting to know my body's rhythm gave me confidence and assurance that I was still on track.

Aside from hormones, I also observed a natural rise and fall of my weight throughout the day and week. Understanding what was "normal" for me was comforting. From morning to night, my weight rises between five to eight pounds, just like clockwork. I could predict Sunday mornings for my lowest weight of the week, and Thursday night my highest. The scale, once hidden in the back of the linen closet, became my most intimate, trusted partner, *my confidential informant*.

I've been so committed to regularly checking my weight that last year on vacation I weighed myself in the hotel lobby every morning—on the luggage scale!

Getting to know my body's fluctuations helped me avoid knee-jerk responses to weight gain. Instead of throwing in the towel, as I would've done in the past after seeing the scale move in the wrong direction, I anticipated and understood what was happening. Knowledge is power! **Befriend the scale and get to know your body's tempo.**

Celebrate (not Sabotage) Success

Keeping track of your progress also gives you the opportunity to document milestones. Celebrating each layer of success is just as important as achieving your goal weight. In fact, I'd like to argue that **the journey is actually the destination.** *That's deep, huh?* Many of us suffer from a false belief that we will only be "good enough" once we reach an arbitrary number on the scale. That couldn't be farther from the truth. Your life is worth celebrating and living to the fullest right now! I would like to proclaim something even more extreme at this point and even suggest that **weight-loss milestones are more meaningful than reaching goal weight! This is actually when the transformation occurs. Milestone celebrations document when behaviors are really changing. Since there technically is no "finish line"** (unless you count death), **the journey is really all you have.**

Prizes and rewards are critical parts of the weight-loss process. On a technical level, they acknowledge and reinforce positive behavioral changes. Who doesn't like a treat? Like Pavlovian dogs, our behavior, both negative and positive, can be manipulated. We don't have to salivate just because a McDonald's jingle starts to play on television. By peppering the journey with positive encouragement, momentum builds. Be creative! Make a chart of mini-goals paired with small rewards you "earn" by losing weight. Think about big and small ways you can pay homage to what you will accomplish. Not only will you set yourself up for success by tracking progress, you will create a visual road map to follow.

If you begin with the end in mind, you are less likely to get lost along the way.

Since I had so much weight to lose, I had a lot to potentially celebrate. (See how I turned being heavy into a positive?) I didn't have a big budget to spend on prizes for myself, but

I still wanted to find meaningful ways to document significant milestones of my weight loss. I seemed to lose about ten pounds a month, so that increment became the focus for commemoration. Starting at ten pounds, twenty pounds, thirty pounds, and so on, I bought a Mylar balloon showing that number, like the kind you buy for a kid's birthday party. Once I lost that number of pounds, my husband would then take a picture of me proudly holding a balloon that celebrated that amount. Looking back at these photos now, I can see my confidence and pride blossoming while my waistline shrunk.

Making progress became contagious. The employees at my local party store got excited when I returned month after

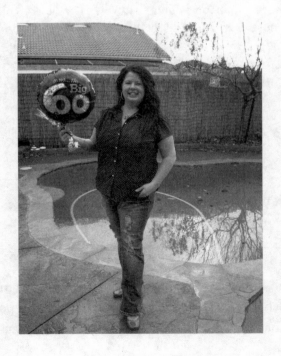

month to buy the next incremental balloon with numbers printed on them: *40, 50, 60, 70, 80, 90, and finally 100!* The 100 mark was the highest available single birthday balloon; from then on, I had to great creative. So, I bought GIANT three-foot-tall individual numbers, *1-1-0, 1-2-0, 1-3-0, 1-4-0!* This whimsical, inexpensive idea was so motivating to my weight loss at the time. I felt special and proud at each separate stage, *not just at the "finish line."* Even now, these photos continue to incentivize me. I wasn't just losing weight in those pictures; I can literally see the emotional growth take place in each incremental photo.

In addition to the balloon celebrations, to hail the "big numbers" along my weight-loss journey, I did what any consumer would do—I cracked open the wallet. When I lost fifty pounds, I bought myself a pair of designer cowboy boots. That decision didn't stem from a love of country music; I was just excited that the *boots finally fit over my calves!* When I reached one hundred pounds of weight lost, I booked a family adventure for horseback riding.

Why? Well, for starters, I would finally have a legitimate reason to wear my cowboy boots. But more important, *because I could.* For the first time in a decade, my weight didn't disqualify me from participating. My weight fell within the permissible guidelines for horseback riding. *Giddyup!*

One might think that buying new clothes would be an obvious reward for weight loss, but for me, this became a financial burden. The expense of replacing my entire wardrobe, almost monthly, was overwhelming. Every ten to fifteen pounds of weight loss meant a full size smaller in clothes. At first, I resisted buying anything new. I continued to wear

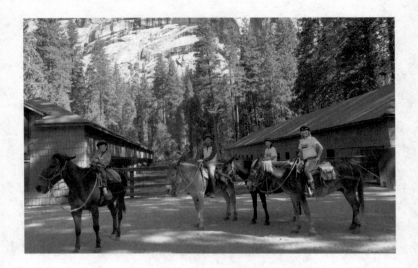

baggy clothes. Sadly, I didn't think I *deserved* a fitted, new wardrobe, as I still believed I weighed "too much." Plus, I had stored boxes of old clothes in my garage that fit me decades ago (musty, out of style, and from the 1980s, no doubt). I was too proud to get rid of those smaller sizes after gaining weight. Instead of buying anything new, I told myself to sift through those unsettling boxes from the back of the garage for something to wear. I should "have" to wear "*those*" clothes, right? My garage clothes turned out to still be too small (*and maybe acid-washed, just sayin'*). It seemed I was in fashion limbo. I decided to just wait.

About this time, I remember struggling to catch a connecting flight at Chicago's O'Hare Airport. To my surprise, my jumbo-sized granny panties were literally *falling off of me*. Rushing through the underground tunnel to reach the terminal, I was pulling my carry-on suitcase with one hand

and holding my underwear up with the other. That embarrassing moment made me rethink my plan to "wait" until I was at goal weight to go shopping.

Out of necessity, I developed a new hobby of shopping at thrift stores. You may turn your nose up at the idea of wearing used clothes, but when you consider the financial cost of replacing a wardrobe not once, not twice, but ELEVEN TIMES in such a short period, you might reconsider. Buying inexpensive clothes at my local Goodwill thrift store helped me transition from one end of the size rack to the other. *That's a lot of clothes, people!* Because the clothes didn't cost very much, I took risks trying out "new looks" for the "new me." The leopard pants might have been a fail (according to my children), but I enjoyed crafting a flamboyant style with vibrant clothes to reflect my emerging confidence.

I even got to know the employees at the thrift stores, since I shopped there so frequently. I developed somewhat of an emotional connection with the workers. Goodwill Industries helps people with barriers to employment by giving them a second chance. I feel like I, too, had been given a second chance at life after losing 140 pounds, so the company's mission statement resonated with me.

Some people might argue you should strap on a hillbilly belt (rope) to your pants and wait until you've reached your goal weight before investing in new clothes. *I couldn't disagree more!* Life continues to happen around you. Work, social events, and everyday activities don't stop just because you have nothing that suitably fits you.

> **Yes, it's superficial, but when you look good,
> you feel better about yourself; higher self-esteem
> leads you to make better choices.**

This is a secret of DIRTY, LAZY, KETO! Whether you buy a few basic pieces or acquire clothes secondhand, don't wait to replace your wardrobe. Correctly sized clothing will flatter your emerging figure and improve your self-esteem. *You are worth the trouble of transitioning to the next size—right now.*

Watch Out for Self-Sabotage

Walking around in a circus tent isn't the only way to thwart progress. Sometimes people think that they are rewarding themselves, but in actuality, their choice of a prize is potentially harmful. ***Perverse rewards*** jeopardize weight-loss success, like eating candy to celebrate losing ten pounds. Be wary of rewards that encourage high-carb eating or of reducing exercise.

Examples of rewards that self-sabotage are in these things we say to ourselves:

- "I lost ten pounds, so I can skip my workout today."
- "I ordered a salad, so I can eat dessert."
- "I've worked so hard; I can take a break while on vacation."
- "Carbs don't count on my birthday!"
- "I went to the gym today, so I can eat that."

How you celebrate incremental weight-loss success is reflective of the outcome you are trying to achieve. That might sound complicated, so let's break it down: having a sundae to celebrate finishing a 5K race reinforces a negative message that you are just running to eat, not eating to run. Running a race doesn't improve an attitude about health if rewarded by junk food. Does that make sense? A more appropriate reward for running a 5K could be purchasing a commemorative headband from the race, or posting bragging rights with finish-line photos on social media, for example. These types of positive rewards reinforce and encourage exercise instead of making you feel sluggish or slothful.

Making consistent healthy decisions is like climbing a set of stairs—each good choice is a step that builds upon the last. Celebrating your achievements, no matter how small or inconsequential they might seem at the time, keeps you moving in the right direction. Incremental celebrations build your confidence and overall feelings of self-worth, giving you the courage to ascend even higher toward your goal.

Hello? The Voice Inside Your Head

We've all heard that staying positive will help us succeed. But when it comes down to it, do you practice this technique? Instead of talking to yourself in a critical voice, your inner thoughts need to be reprogrammed to provide encouragement. By hearing only positive internal messages of self-love, you can coach yourself to become a winner who believes you deserve to be at goal weight.

One of the standout memories from my own weight-loss journey that supports this belief occurred during an unexpected breakdown in a Kohl's fitting room. I'm not a crier at all; in fact, I consider myself to be the opposite. As a proud, dysfunctional midwesterner, I swallow my emotions stoically, *often accompanied with food.* I think that's why this public display of emotion was so memorable to me.

When you're "morbidly" obese, you tend to shop mostly online. There are only a handful of physical stores that sell larger sizes. I happen to live in a semirural area, so my selection of stores was pretty limited to begin with. My discount options were Walmart or Ross, and if I was feeling fancy, upscale options were JCPenney, Kohl's, or Macy's. Welcome to small-town America!

Because I had an upcoming "business casual" event spring up on my calendar, I ventured out to my local department store to buy a decent pair of jeans that fit. I had received a ten-dollar-off coupon in the mail for Kohl's department store, and that motivated me to explore uncharted waters. I hadn't bought a pair of jeans in YEARS. I found the fabric to be unforgiving to my ever-expanding size, and I preferred pants with an elastic waist. Plus (*sorry, no pun intended*), the boring designs of size 26 jeans usually looked like "mom jeans," if you know what I mean.

After perusing the plain and boring options from the plus-size department, I grabbed one of each style from sizes toward the end of the rack. Surely, since I had lost "some weight," I hoped at least one of these drab pants would fit. Boy, was I in for a surprise!

The 26 and 24 size jeans were remarkably too big. In fact, after zipping them up (usually a feat that occurred only by my lying flat on the bed), I could still slide them off over my hips. Like MC Hammer, I danced around the fitting room shaking my parachute-pants butt with amusement. If the 24 and 26 pants were too big, then what size might actually fit? A mess of clothing from a previous shopper was piled high in the corner of my dressing room—an innocent pair of size 18 Levi's laid on top. On a whim, before my mind could protect me from the potential despair that might follow, I yanked them off the hanger and started pulling them on.

Oh, sweet Jesus—they fit. They FIT! THEY FIT!

My eyes welled up with tears, and for a moment I couldn't breathe. Not because the pants were too tight, but the size 18 tag stunned me. I don't think I ever wore a size 18 before! Somehow, in the blink of the eye, I had gone from an everyday high schooler wearing junior-size jeans from the mall to an extremely obese adult with a wardrobe of only unflattering elastic.

Yet here I was, at the finest department store in my rural town, wearing SIZE 18 JEANS!

With tears running down my face, I stuck my hips out, one at a time, admiring my apparent figure in the mirror. I laughed and smiled at my childlike response. "Brooke Shields, WATCH OUT!" I thought, and for just one fleeting moment, *all the negative voices inside my head were silenced.*

This standout memory from my weight-loss journey was about more than just shopping. This was a turning point in my confidence. "I can do this. This is working. I AM doing this!" went through my mind. I cried happy tears onto that fitting room floor with a flimsy bathroom lock protecting my fragile emotional state. The pride I felt in that moment tasted better than any buttered popcorn. *I was hooked.*

Non-Scale Victories

Buying those Levi's marked the first of many "non-scale victories" (NSVs) I celebrated along my weight-loss trek. Perhaps more important than a number on the scale, NSVs improved my emotional confidence. I wanted to collect them like badges on a Girl Scout sash. I was winning small battles. The amount I weighed paled in comparison to how non-scale victories made me feel. *I felt strong and powerful.*

Other standout memories worth noting:

- Seeing my C-section scar *for the first time* without using a mirror.
- Fitting into my husband's T-shirt.
- Shopping for a bra at Victoria's Secret (*a normal people's store!*).
- Having my wedding rings resized not once, but TWICE!
- Changing the seat adjustments in my car because my stomach no longer hit the steering wheel.
- Realizing all my shoes were too big (my shoe size dropped a full size).
- Sitting comfortably in a movie theater seat.
- Painting my own toenails.
- Taking a nap on the couch (not using a recliner, but the long way).
- Participating in my son's T-ball games.
- The first time I noticed someone "checking me out."
- Easily clasping a seat belt on an airplane (That NEVER gets old!).

FACEBOOK SHOUT-OUTS

Non-Scale Victories from the DLK Support Group:

"My toddler and I fit comfortably in this chair together. We're snuggling for the first time!" —Brittany

"I have type 2 diabetes and my doctor just told me to stop all my meds!" —Mia

"Within a week I lost my sweet tooth. I'm shocked!" —Park

"I just shaved my bikini line without lifting my stomach up!" —Vanessa

"I fit in the booth at Applebee's." —Sarah

"I picked up my husband today at work. It was raining, so I didn't want to get out of the car. I climbed over the center console into the passenger seat to open the door. I couldn't believe I could do that!" —Emily

"I have to get my class ring resized." —Chen

"I went to the water park with my family today. I pranced around the whole park in a swimsuit. I felt CONFIDENT!" —Angelica

"My A1C is now 4.9!" —Melody

"My husband just bought a new belt. He ran out of holes to make it smaller." —Sandy

"Today I bought size 14 jeans; not impressed? I used to wear size 50!" —Erin

3

I'M NOT SUPPOSED TO EAT THAT!

Work with Yourself, Not Against

I read an article recently that labeled the keto diet as a "last resort." I felt as if I were slapped. I took offense to those words because calling keto "last resort" implies this way of eating is not advisable or, even worse, unsafe. Nothing gets me more fired up than hearing this type of ignorant criticism. Why is everyone so judgmental about how other people eat? This is a topic that my best friend, Tamara, and I like to discuss while walking our dogs. Not only is Tamara hilarious, but she often makes me yell, "HUH!" (like, "*Wow*, I never thought of that!"), both important qualities when choosing an exercise partner.

"Diets are the new religion," she stated. "People identify with a group of like-minded eaters and follow 'rules' as if they were doctrine."

That's a controversial statement with bold kernels of truth. We all want to fit in somewhere. Being part of a group makes us feel safe and "right." Having established rules keeps order and harmony. That's all good, right? Not so fast. Sometimes being part of a group leads to self-righteousness. When this happens, people condemn anyone "not" in their group, proclaiming their own practices as superior. Let me share a mild example.

I have a very thin neighbor who absolutely loves the Weight Watchers program. She tries to goad me into keto fights whenever we bump into each other at school events.

"I brought Corn Nuts for the classroom snack because *I don't* have a problem with carbs," she quipped, with a snide smile and tilt of the head. "Want some?"

Instead of being irritated, I found her childlike behavior amusing. I couldn't care less about the Corn Nuts (*though they do give her bad breath, just sayin'*), but I am bothered by the subtle message being insinuated: *I'm better than you because I'm not limited with my food choices.* Her behavior is not uncommon. People spend their whole lives inside a bubble, convinced they are right about everything. They believe their way is the only way, without compassion or a willingness to believe there are other ways of doing things. Hmmm . . . *WHY IS THAT?*

Keto Police

Even within the keto community, splinter groups conflict. Evangelical keto police take great pride in calling out straying members of their own tribe, shouting "THAT'S NOT

KETO!" to anyone caught sipping a Diet Coke. You might laugh, but keto vigilantes push their beliefs to the extreme. They ridicule, block, and name-call fellow ketonians, all in the name of self-perceived *keto righteousness*. As the host of a large Facebook group, I have a front-row seat to these arguments. I've witnessed a fruitful debate over the merits of coffee creamer escalate into ugly catfights with profanity, threats, and ultimatums being issued. Because I see this behavior happen so often, I worry. I struggle to understand why mature, *grown-ass* men and women stoop to such low levels just to "be right." Aren't we in this together? Shouldn't we support one another instead of tearing one another down?

Why do bullies ridicule, anyway? I know there is absolutely no valid excuse for taunting and teasing, but I'm still curious why it happens. Is a bully's fragile ego just trying to protect itself? By making other people feel small, bullies shine a bold spotlight away from themselves. They scream so loudly at others hoping no one looks back toward their direction. Through criticism and ranting, I suspect keto bullies are trying to hide their own vulnerability or weakness.

The truth is that we are all scared. Many of us really may not know completely what we are doing when it comes to eating healthy. We've been told to *not eat this* and definitely *not that,* for our entire lives; we may all be confused about which foods are "right" or "wrong" to eat. Weight loss seems like a mystery. Popular wisdom about cholesterol, fat, and calories revises its position every decade. We are terrified to admit it, but NO ONE seems to have *all* of the answers. Every single one of us at times feels insecure about what to do, including me! If only we would lower our guards and admit to feeling vulnerable. Maybe then we could start helping and not hurting one another while we try to figure this out.

Breaking Myths About Dieting

For years, I didn't tell anyone how I lost weight. Instead of risking an argument about whether my food choices were nutritionally sound, I remained silent. The truth is that I probably couldn't have defended myself properly at the time. I felt like the way I lost weight was by doing something wrong. Who eats sour cream and goes down eleven pants sizes? It seemed *biologically suspicious*. Growing up, I listened to my family doctor insisting I had to eat low-fat foods and restrict calories to lose weight, but here I was as a grown-up, eating cheese and bacon, never feeling hungry, and yet losing weight. Surely I was doing something "illegal." It's taken me years to build up enough courage to talk about this stuff.

The key reason I think I've been successful with losing weight is that **I finally figured out what worked for me and *not* everybody else.** I stopped trying to be the kind of eater the world wanted me to become. I reevaluated dieting "truths" by asking myself if they still made sense to me. For my entire life, I've been told how I *should eat*. In the end, I had to throw out that rule book for me to lose weight.

Senseless Guidelines I Disobey

- Fat is bad for you.
- Never eat in front of the television.
- You must limit your calories.
- Eat only when you're hungry.
- Always choose nonfat or low-fat foods.
- Eat slowly.
- Desserts are bad for you.
- Don't snack between meals.
- Breakfast is the most important meal of the day.
- Fast food is unhealthy.
- Ladies order salads.
- Never have seconds.
- Oatmeal is the ideal breakfast food.
- Fried foods cause high cholesterol.
- Girls shouldn't eat that much.
- Don't use food to cover up your feelings.
- No snacking after dinner.
- Eat foods that "stick to your ribs," like rice or pasta.
- Eggs cause high cholesterol.
- Weight loss and hunger go hand in hand.
- You can't eat desserts and lose weight at the same time.

I've learned that by challenging these weight-loss myths, I could rewrite new truths. I like to eat while watching television, so *sue me*! Who says eating and relaxing have to be separate activities? Who really cares if I eat seconds at dinner? *No one is keeping score.* Instead of feeling like crap about myself for eating fast food or munching on a snack before dinner, I decided to say, ENOUGH!

I've finally broken the cycle of guilt, inadequacy, and shame that led me to constantly overeat. Instead of disappointing myself by constantly not meeting expectations, I'm consciously walking away from these silly notions altogether. I'm never going to be a dainty, ladylike eater who "just orders a salad." I would feel unsatisfied! I prefer to eat large portions of food, and if I'm laying it all out here, I will admit to eating frequently, as well. I decided to do what worked for me and nobody else.

#BreakTheRules

I needed to break away from society's judgment and expectations to lose weight on my own terms.

Working with my personality, and not against, is liberating. Because there are no "rules" to follow, I find myself being more honest. **I don't cheat because there are no rules to cheat against.** I created a new set of personal values and have figured out the types of foods that support my new lifestyle.

To make this work, I had to be honest with myself. I had to ask introspective questions like these:

- How much accountability do I need?
- If I don't write down everything I eat, will I be proud of my choices?
- Will documenting my food in a tracker *help* or *detract* from making better food choices?

Some people depend on food diaries for success. They lose more weight when they honestly document their meals (on paper or with an app). There are definite advantages to keeping a tracker, but it doesn't mean it's the only "right way." The theory is that if you have to record every bite, you might think twice about shoving it in your mouth. It's a system of accountability or means of enforcement. If writing things down works for you, then I say go for it! I have a colleague who enjoys the MyFitnessPal app and digitally records her meals into her smartphone. It works well with her personality. For me, being chained to an app would be *torture*. The bottom line is, do what works for you and your personality.

Rebels like me bristle at this kind of tracking, preferring instead a less restrictive approach. I mentally keep a tally of how many net carbs I eat each day, with the goal of staying within a range of 20–50 grams of net carbs. While I was losing weight, my losses were sometimes volatile due to inaccuracies in my tracking method. I wasn't cheating, mind you, just a bit remiss sometimes about staying within my range. I decided that consequence was okay with me. I've been forced to use trackers in the past by counting points with Weight Watchers, and I found them super irritating, like an annoying task on a "to-do list." I didn't want to resent my new lifestyle by drowning myself with busywork. I wanted to avoid any useless or painful tasks that would cause me to rebel, cheat, or, worse, *quit*.

#BreakTheRules

My goal was to adopt permanent lifestyle changes. I wanted to lose my weight and keep it off *for-evah*. I needed to retrain my brain to make consistent choices to achieve this goal. It worked! I am committed to making the right choices independently. For me, I predicted a food tracker would have caused me more harm than good, and I was right. Call me juvenile, but hand me a little report card to fill out about my eating, and I will immediately start looking for loophole opportunities to cheat. Just like maxing out a credit card, I knew a tracker would also allow me to overeat net carbs one day with the hope of paying for it in the future. I couldn't depend on a tracker as my long-term solution. I needed to go at it on my own.

Does counting carbs have to be all one way or another? Absolutely not. One of the benefits of DIRTY, LAZY, KETO is that it is flexible to your individual needs and lifestyle. If I notice my weight has started to creep up, I have the option of returning to a stricter version until my weight gets back under control. I recognize the value and importance of being accountable to myself with my eating. I am willing to be "irritated" with the task of writing down my food choices for a couple weeks if that means I can then easily put on my Miss Me jeans without having to lay back on the bed and suck in my gut to zip them up. Whether you document calories, macros, net carbs, or a combination thereof, choose a method that is effective, yet comfortable for you to continue long-term. Your method has to be practical yet bearable for this to work. Ultimately, DIRTY, LAZY, KETO becomes your lifestyle.

I Can Eat Anything I Want!

My friend Sarah also lost over a hundred pounds eating a DIRTY, LAZY, KETO diet and has kept her weight off for several years. When asked to share her personal strategy for successful weight-loss maintenance, she replied, "I know what foods I can eat, and I just eat those foods." Like Sarah, you can make accountability as simple as you desire, or as complex. By being consistent, you will be successful!

I often remind myself that *no food is off-limits*. This is a reframing technique I use to trick myself. Yes, this might sound childish, but it's really effective. Instead of complaining about the foods I "can't" eat, I convince myself that *I'm choosing what foods to eat*. I think it's a mental thing, like shunning the forbidden fruit. If a food is important enough, I figure out a way to make a DLK substitute. I have yet to find a food that doesn't have a low-carb alternative that still satisfies me. Especially with desserts, there is always a way to make a recipe sugar-free. I don't turn my nose up at artificial sugars; instead, I embrace and appreciate their help.

Your physical cravings for sweets will drastically decrease as you become fat-adapted. Over time, even your sense of smell will improve. I can smell the stench of sugar from across the room. *(It's kind of freaky!)* Old habits and emotional triggers for sweets, on the other hand, *don't* change overnight. Those triggers take hard work to address and can't be fixed so easily. In the meantime, I suggest having "safe" sweet substitutes on hand to help get you through those moments when you MUST HAVE SOMETHING SWEET RIGHT THIS SECOND!

Judge if you want to, but sugar alcohols have been my savior. Notice I didn't say sugar *and* alcohol—*ha!* If you don't understand what sugar alcohols are, you're not alone. Sugar alcohols are reduced-calorie sweeteners, but they do not contain alcohol. *Okayyyyyyyy????* So why do we care? Well, sugar alcohols are used more and more in reduced-calorie foods. Sugar substitutes are common in keto-substitution products, like Halo Top ice cream. When I need to, I splurge on keto sweet treats, such as sugar-free chocolates, hard candy, and protein bars, more affectionately known as "candy bars in drag."

Though they do not contribute to tooth decay like normal table sugar does, sugar alcohols can have foul effects on your digestive system when eaten beyond the recommended serving size. Bloating, flatulence, and uncontrollable diarrhea are possible unpleasant side effects. *That's really disgusting,* so indulge with caution.

Whenever I'm at a work meeting, invariably antsy and sucking away on sugar-free candy, some unprepared soul will ask me for a piece. Depending on how well I like the person, I'll share my candy (with or without warning them first!). Some folks experience nasty gastrointestinal consequences after eating a single-serving dose of sugar-free candy, while others, who possess a bulletproof constitution, are fine.

I've definitely had heated arguments with fellow dieting friends about the role sugar substitutes should play in how we prepare foods. They argue that these chemicals are harmful and recommend to "just cut back" or substitute a more natural source of sugar instead like agave, honey, or maple syrup. I've learned to smile politely when I hear these ridiculous suggestions (*while inside my head screaming*), "DON'T YOU THINK I'VE TRIED THAT ALREADY?"

Obviously, I have to agree that eating chemically processed fake sugar probably isn't good for me (to put it mildly). But after much consideration, I've decided to take my chances.

This argument reminds me of a scene in the movie *A Few Good Men* (1992), in which Jack Nicholson yells, "You can't handle the truth!" That's how I feel about any natural cousins of my evil sugar nemesis: *"Stephanie, you can't handle the sugar!"*

I'm certain that eating sugar, in any of its forms, will lead me back on the path to weight gain—*I guarantee it*. I'm just one vending-machine trip away to starting to regain 140 pounds—*sugar is THAT addictive to me!* Instead, I'm choosing step-down therapy—Splenda, monk fruit, *whatever*! But NOT sugar. DIRTY, LAZY, KETO supports the use of sugar substitutes to help you break the sugar-addicted cause of obesity, even those substitutes that are chemically or artificially processed. Sometimes you have to pick your poison. Instead of shopping in the plus size department, I choose Splenda. I empower you to make your own choice, too, *without* any judgment or criticism.

How to Manage a Sweet Tooth

My sweet tooth perks up in three distinct situations. First, I notice that I will crave something sweet if my last meal was *unexpectedly too high* in carbs (resulting in a crash of blood sugar). This can happen when I'm not 100 percent sure what ingredients are in a dish, like when I eat at a buffet or at a friend's house. You can research only so much; sometimes, a problematic food slips under your radar. It can be scary when I unknowingly eat too many carbs, because all of a sudden I'm craving sugar like an addict.

Early in my weight-loss journey, my husband was trying to be supportive by making "something healthy" for dinner. I gobbled up the delicious keto chili he made from a recipe he had found online. I trusted that it was "safe" because the word "low-carb" were in the title. I ate two large bowls and praised his cooking. *Yummy!* About a half hour or so after dinner, however, I started having insane sugar cravings. I was freaking out! I investigated the recipe further. Chickpeas, crushed tomatoes, black beans, and tomato paste were among the offending ingredients. No wonder my body was going into glucose overload!

I've learned to push through sweet-tooth cravings instead of giving in, weathering the storm, so to speak. Interestingly, I've found that walking outside or drinking salty broth (that sounds fancy but can be as simple as a bouillon cube mixed with hot water) helps curb the cravings faster. Also, if I'm feeling really stressed out, I notice I'll start to crave something sweet. *I'm human, remember?* Since eating sugar or anything sweet releases dopamine, it makes sense that my body craves sugar as an antidote. Lastly, I have a habit of eating something sweet after I finish dinner. That's not a physical need, it's just a habit. I don't fight this urge; instead, I plan for a sugar-free treat.

Acknowledging and honoring my sweet tooth helps me to be successful. Instead of running from the cravings, I plan for them. For example, I enjoy a sweet snack as my dessert immediately following dinner (not hours later). DIRTY, LAZY, KETO daily dessert rituals I rely on are sugar-free Jell-O sometimes topped with a squirt of real whipped cream, sugar-free chocolates, and caffeine-free, artificially flavored tea. If I'm in the mood for a pastry, I might toast a high-fiber tortilla topped with butter, cinnamon, and Splenda for a "churro" type treat.

Berries are a staple in my kitchen: blueberries, strawberries, or raspberries equal low-carb deliciousness when enjoyed in moderation. For an even more luxurious treat, I top the berries with a splash of half-and-half stirred with a zero net carbs sweetener.

**As my husband always says,
"Berries are truly nature's candy!"**

If I'm feeling fancy, I have been known to serve berries with mascarpone (rich Italian cream cheese blended with sugar substitute and vanilla flavoring). For special holidays, I make a low-carb cheesecake. I don't eat rich desserts too often, because I have a hard time stopping myself. Even though I don't keep track of calories, common sense tells me not to make cheesecake too frequently. It's better for me to have a little sugar-free Jell-O versus a slice of cheesecake, even if both desserts are low in net carbs.

> **Planning to indulge your sweet tooth doesn't mean
> you're a failure at losing weight. On the contrary,
> it makes you a DIRTY, LAZY, KETO hero!**

The Snack Attack

You don't have to give up sweets or stop snacking while losing weight on DIRTY, LAZY, KETO. I'm going to say out loud what no one wants to admit. If you're anything like me, your habits are unlikely to change! There, I said it. I'm tired of trying to "fix myself." For my entire life, I've tried (and failed) to create healthier routines like cutting out desserts or not eating between meals. I've got news for ya—*this ain't gonna happen!*

When I first get home from work, I have an instant "snack attack." I walk into the kitchen and grab something to eat. Whether I'm hungry or not isn't the issue; I do this out of habit. I usually start snacking and continue snacking all the way until I eat dinner. I remember (in my previous life), a Weight Watchers counselor suggested that instead of coming directly home from work, I should go to the gym, or perhaps take a walk to avoid the "witching hour of snacking." I appreciated her suggestion, but deep down, I didn't *really* want to change that habit. Perhaps in a perfect world I would go to the gym every day, but the truth is that kind of schedule switch is unrealistic for me. I'm too tired! I don't want to set myself up for failure by expecting drastic changes like that.

Sometimes you have to admit the truth, and my truth is that *I like to snack to relax.*

Since it's unlikely I'm going to change my snacking habits, I decided to stop fighting this pattern of behavior and work with my current habits. *If I'm going to snack, snack, snack, then I need to substitute, substitute, substitute.* To make my snacking even more complicated to manage, I'm also a voluminous eater. (Doesn't that sound like a breed of dinosaur?) This means I unknowingly eat until I'm past the point of being full. *(Boy, that's a little embarrassing, even for me to admit!)*

I've learned that there are foods I can eat in large quantities without derailing my weight loss. Cruciferous vegetables are my go-to companion. The fiber eventually fills the void that chips previously tried to fill. When topped with a healthy fat, low carb veggies are my secret weight-loss weapon.

Depending on how voracious my hunger is during a snack attack, here are some of my "go-to" favorites:

- Artichoke leaves dipped in mayo
- Cauliflower "faux" potatoes
- Celery with nut butter
- Jalapeño poppers
- Olives
- Pickles
- Raw cauliflower with dip
- Salads with a creamy dressing like Blue Cheese
- Vegetable soup
- Zucchini spears dipped in Ranch dressing

Comforting Foods

In autumn, when the weather cools, my body transitions from wanting summer "crunchy" type foods to craving the comfort foods of fall. I grew up in the Midwest with long cold winters, and my family survived the cold with a staple of lasagnas, casseroles, and hearty soups. Colder weather makes me crave the comfort and simplicity of my childhood. During my weight-loss journey, I noticed weather changes affected my eating. When it was cold and rainy outside, I wanted to eat warm foods in large quantities.

I have found more success in working with, not against, these desires. *Modify, modify, modify.* I updated my childhood favorite recipes to include more fats, a moderate amount of protein, but with drastically reduced net carbs. With my Crock-Pot keeping refills warm, I enjoy bowl after bowl of a creamy soup or hearty stew. I don't feel an ounce of guilt pulling an overflowing tray of low-carb lasagna out of the oven for dinner (use whole milk ricotta or cottage cheese 4 percent milkfat* and a noodle substitute like zucchini). I figured out how to enjoy my favorite meals without causing my blood sugar levels to go unchecked. By increasing the non-starchy, cruciferous vegetables (for added fiber) in the recipe and including favorite fats (healthy oils, full-fat dairy cheese, sour cream, or yogurt), I've successfully adapted familiar comfort recipes to earn a passing grade from DIRTY, LAZY, KETO.[†]

---

* Cottage cheese, 4% milkfat, 5 g net carbs per ½ cup serving
† Shameless plug here: You'll love the homespun recipes included in *The DIRTY, LAZY, KETO Cookbook: Bend the Rules to Lose the Weight!* by Stephanie and William Laska (Simon & Schuster, 2020).

Bell Pepperoni Pizza Cup

Yield: 6 servings ⟩ Prep time: 10 minutes ⟩ Cook time: 35 minutes ⟩ 5 net carbs/serving

I love recipes that sneak in vegetables when I'm least expecting it. These bell peppers, when filled with traditional pizza toppings, make me think I'm eating pepperoni pizza!

INGREDIENTS

3 medium green bell peppers, halved from top to bottom, cored and seeded

8 tablespoons olive oil, divided

¾ cup no-sugar-added marinara sauce

1 cup shredded mozzarella cheese

1 cup shredded cheddar cheese

¼ cup sliced black olives

1 teaspoon minced jalapeño

1 tablespoon chopped white onion

¼ cup sliced mushrooms

18 slices pepperoni

⅛ teaspoon salt

⅛ teaspoon red pepper flakes

2 tablespoons Parmesan cheese

DIRECTIONS

1. Preheat oven to 375°F.
2. In a large, microwave-safe dish, microwave bell pepper halves on high for 4 minutes.
3. Use 2 tablespoons oil to grease bottom of 9×13-inch glass baking dish.

4. Distribute bell peppers evenly like boats, open side facing up.

5. Fill each bell pepper with 1 tablespoon oil, 2 tablespoons marinara sauce.

6. Distribute mozzarella and cheddar cheeses evenly over each bell pepper.

7. Top bell peppers with pizza toppings: olives, jalapeños, onions, mushrooms, and pepperoni.

8. Sprinkle salt, red pepper flakes, and Parmesan cheese evenly over peppers.

9. Cover with aluminum foil and bake 30 minutes. Remove foil and bake 5 minutes or until cheese browns.

Skeletal Chicken Soup

Yield: 8 servings ⟩ Prep time: 20 minutes ⟩ Cook time: 70 minutes ⟩ 2 net carbs/serving

Do you remember eating Campbell's Chicken & Stars soup as a child? The softened, riced cauliflower in this recipe tastes similar to those pasta-shaped stars from our childhood favorite. Eating Skeletal Chicken Soup provides a nostalgic feeling of coming inside to warm up after playing in the snow. As a result, this soup fills me up, both emotionally and physically.

If you're in a hurry, skip making the broth from scratch (this is lazy keto, right?). Open up a can of broth or pop a couple of bouillon cubes into hot water; I won't tell! If you haven't tried making bone broth from scratch before, though, let me convince you that it's worth the effort. You can even stash a leftover rotisserie-chicken carcass in your freezer for this occasion. Cooking broth from scratch will make your house smell absolutely amazing, and you can waltz around the kitchen like Julia Child. Additionally, similar to pickle juice, bone broth replenishes electrolytes.

INGREDIENTS

1 rotisserie chicken

¼ cup olive oil

1 cup diced celery

1 small carrot, finely chopped

2 cups riced cauliflower (purchase frozen—already riced; or fresh—rice it by hand using a grater or food processor)

1 cup sliced zucchini

½ cup thinly sliced mushrooms

¼ cup chopped green onion

¼ cup finely chopped fresh herbs: equal parts of parsley, rosemary, and thyme

1 teaspoon salt

½ teaspoon pepper

DIRECTIONS

1. Remove chicken meat from rotisserie chicken. Set meat aside.

2. In a large soup pot, cover carcass with 8 cups water. Bring to boil, simmer 60 minutes (or longer, if you have the time).

3. In separate, large skillet, heat oil using medium heat and sauté celery and carrots until softened. Set aside.

4. Strain chicken stock: remove and dispose bones and cartilage. Return broth to soup pot.

5. Add pulled chicken meat, oil, vegetables, herbs, and spices to pot of broth.

6. Cover and return to boil. Reduce temperature to low and simmer for 10 minutes, stirring regularly. Serve warm.

Cravings for Salt, Sugar, and Fat

The effect that the seasons and weather have over your mood is well-documented; many people suffer from depression throughout the winter months. Feeling blue can lead to over-eating. If you are like me and you historically gain weight during the winter, spending time preparing comforting meals can make or break your weight-loss plans. Whether food cravings are sparked by outside influences like the temperature, or from inside your body like with hormone changes, recognizing eating patterns is the first step.

Gentlemen, feel free to skip to the next section. Ladies, you know what I'm going to talk about here. Prior to your monthly cycle, do you notice that you crave foods higher in salt, sugar, and/or fat? In my previous life, I never paid attention to changes in my cravings. I ate sugary, salty, fattening foods twenty-four seven! Once I started DIRTY, LAZY, KETO, however, I started to notice patterns. I observed a marked change in my eating behaviors just prior to the start of my period. Additionally, I noted my weight would artificially inflate at that same time but then drop back down once my period was over. It took a few months of patient observation to figure out this pattern.

When you're trying to lose weight, even the slightest gain causes panic. You might overreact and be tempted to quit. Predicting my weight fluctuations and being prepared when they occurred was such an important lesson to learn. In my previous weight-loss experiences, an upswing in my weight could prompt me to fall off the wagon and simply give up. Now, I'm aware of these patterns and not thrown off course when my body screams for sweets, chocolate, or fried foods. I'm kicking myself that it took so long for me to figure this out.

Now that I'm more aware of my body's demands during this time of the month, I feel more prepared and in control. I actually keep "supplies" on hand in case of food-craving emergencies. For chocolate cravings, some of my "go-to" options include:

- Avocado Chocolate Pudding*
- Cacao 100% unsweetened baking chocolate, 1 g net carb per 2 piece (14 gram) serving
- Cacao 85–86% chocolate, 6 g net carbs per 2.5 pieces (30 gram) serving
- Cacao 92% chocolate, 6 g net carbs per 3 pieces (34 gram) serving
- Cacao powder (cocoa powder) 100% unsweetened, 1 g net carb per 1 tablespoon serving
- Cocoa roasted almonds, 3 g net carbs per 1 (17.5 gram) packet
- Chocolate Cake Batter (recipe provided)
- Chocolate candy,[†] varies according to brand, estimated 1–2 g net carb per 2–5 piece serving
- Chocolate chips (sugar-free, sweetened with *malitol*[‡]), 8 g net carbs per 1 tablespoon serving
- Chocolate chips (sugar-free, sweetened with *stevia*[§]), 1 g net carb per 60 chip (14 gram) serving

---

* Secret Ingredient Chocolate Pudding from *The DIRTY, LAZY, KETO Cookbook: Bend the Rules to Lose the Weight!* by Stephanie and William Laska (Simon & Schuster, 2020)
† Russell Stover Assorted Sugar-free Chocolates, Hershey's Sugar-free Chocolate
‡ Hershey's Kitchens Baking Chips
§ Lily's Sweets

- Chocolate Icy (recipe provided)
- Chocolate snack bar (Atkins), 2–4 g net carbs per 1 (1.4 oz.) bar
- Chocolate syrup, sugar-free, 1 g net carb per 1 tablespoon serving
- Cinnamon Mocha Coffee (recipe provided)
- Double Chocolate Chunk protein bar (Quest), 4 g net carbs per 1 (2.12 oz.) bar (60 gram) serving
- Hot cocoa (nonfat powdered mix with water), 4 g net carbs per (8 gram) envelope serving*
- Ice cream, chocolate (low-carb†), varies per brand, estimated 0–1 g net carb per ½ cup serving

Fried Foods

If I'm not craving sweets at a certain time of the month, next in line is a strong desire for salty FRIED FOODS. French fries, potato poppers, jalapeño poppers, chicken strips, fried mozzarella sticks . . . You name it, I'll crave it! Basically, anything you might find on an appetizer menu is on my wish list when I'm premenstrual. Hormonal cravings for high-carb foods don't go away just because you are eating DIRTY, LAZY, KETO. Instead of driving to happy hour, I've found at-home alternatives that satisfy me (or at least trick my brain). It's easy to enjoy fried foods on DIRTY, LAZY, KETO. In lieu of

---

* Nonfat powdered hot chocolate ironically has fewer carbs than the sugar-free variety and has about 4 g of net carbs per serving. I can stretch that packet into two servings to get more carb bang for the buck.
† Popular low-carb brands of ice cream: Enlightened, Halo Top, Rebel

breading your meat or vegetable with white flour or buttermilk, coat using a lower carb flour substitute. Fry or bake to a crisp and dip in ranch dressing. *You're welcome!*

The bottom line is that you need to become aware of your body's cycle and work with it, not against it. You are unlikely to solve the riddle of premenstrual agitation for women around the world, but you may discover how to manage your own cravings when they arrive by being prepared with higher fat, low-carb, moderate protein options.

DIRTY, LAZY, KETO Flour Substitutes*

Almond flour (super-fine), 3 g net carbs per ¼ cup serving

Carbquik Baking Mix, 2 g net carbs per ⅓ cup serving

Coconut flour, 4–5 net carbs per ¼ cup serving

Flaxseed (ground), 1 g net carb per 2 tablespoon serving

Flaxseed meal (whole), 2 g net carb per 2½ tablespoon serving

Hemp seeds (shelled), 1 g net carbs per 3 tablespoon serving

Parmesan cheese, 0 g carb per 1 teaspoon serving

Pork rinds, 0 g net carbs per 1 oz. serving

Psyllium husk powder, 1 g net carb per 1 teaspoon serving

Soy flour, 5 g net carbs per ¼ cup serving

Vital wheat gluten flour, 1 g net carb per 1 tablespoon serving

---

* Only for reference: Note that all-purpose enriched white flour has 84 g net carbs per 1 cup serving and all-natural whole wheat flour follows close behind with 72 g net carbs per 1 cup serving.

Recipes for Sweet and Fried Cravings

I'll share with you some of my favorite recipes—chocolate, sweet, and fried—that have helped me weather precarious moments of intense cravings.

Chocolate Icy

Yield: 1 serving ⟩ Prep time: 3 minutes ⟩ Cook time: 0 minutes ⟩ 3 net carbs/serving

When a chocolate craving hits, my blender is armed and ready to serve. In under three minutes, I can create a Chocolate Icy drink better than any Frosty from Wendy's.

INGREDIENTS
2 cups ice
¼ cup half-and-half
2 tablespoons unsweetened cocoa powder
1 cup unsweetened almond milk
8 packets of zero net carbs sweetener

DIRECTIONS
Add all ingredients to blender. Pulse for 60 seconds until desired consistency is reached. Pour into tall malt glasses and enjoy with a spoon or straw.

Cinnamon Mocha Coffee

Yield: 1 serving ⟩ Prep time: 3 minutes ⟩ Cook Time: 0 minutes ⟩ 2 net carbs/serving

I prefer to create elaborate coffees in my kitchen in lieu of handing over my hard-earned cash to Starbucks. My Cinnamon Mocha Coffee recipe is light on net carbs but heavy on taste. And I can enjoy this without changing out of my pajamas!

INGREDIENTS

1 cup freshly brewed hot coffee

2 tablespoons (full-fat) half-and-half

1 teaspoon unsweetened cocoa powder

¼ teaspoon vanilla (real or imitation)

2 packets zero net carbs sweetener

Cinnamon stick

Dash of salt

DIRECTIONS

In a coffee mug, blend all ingredients using immersion blender (or small glass blender suited for blending hot liquids). Serve in coffee mug with cinnamon stick. *Enjoy!*

Chocolate Cake Batter

Yield: 1 serving ⟩ Prep time: 3 minutes ⟩ Cook time: 0 minutes ⟩ 6 net carbs/serving

I prefer to start the day with something sweet and scandalous. Sadly, I've never been a fan of a "healthy" breakfast. In fact, I spent most of my adult life choosing a colorful Danish to start my day. Instead of fighting my urge for something sweet when I wake up, I often treat myself to Chocolate Cake Batter for breakfast, topped with chocolate chips, and licked off a spatula, to boot!

INGREDIENTS

1 cup 5% milk fat Greek strained yogurt

1 teaspoon unsweetened cocoa powder

¼ teaspoon vanilla (pure or imitation)

3 packets zero net carbs sweetener

1 tablespoon sugar-free chocolate chips (sweetened with
   stevia)

DIRECTIONS

In a small bowl, blend yogurt with cocoa powder, vanilla, and
   sweetener.

Top with chocolate chips and serve cold.

Orange Push-Pop

Yield: 1 serving ⟩ Prep time: 3 minutes ⟩ Cook time: 0 minutes ⟩ 2 net
carbs/serving

*Nostalgic summer memories of buying Push-Ups from the ice
cream truck fueled my desire to replicate this fruity, hot-weather
snack. I am so obsessed with this quick, low-calorie orange dessert that I now order sugar-free gelatin boxes by the case from
Amazon!*

INGREDIENTS

2 cups ice

3 tablespoons (full-fat) half-and-half

1 (12 fl. oz.) can diet orange soda

1 small box sugar-free orange gelatin powder (.32 oz. or .30 oz.
   depending on brand)

Add all ingredients to blender.

Cover and pulse for 60 seconds until desired consistency is reached.

(Start slowly, as orange soda is carbonated and may foam up.)

Pour into a tall glass and enjoy with a wide straw.

Jumpin' Jicama Fries

Yield: 5 servings 〉 Prep time: 10 minutes 〉 Cook time: 30–40 minutes 〉
5 net carbs/serving

Peeling a jicama is no joke. Once that arduous task is completed, the real challenge begins—cutting the jicama fries to precisely the same shape. Not only will this help the fries cook evenly, but your brain will be fooled into thinking you hit the drive-thru.

INGREDIENTS

1 medium jicama, peeled, trimmed, and evenly cut into desired fry
    shapes

¼ cup olive oil

½ cup Parmesan cheese

⅛ teaspoon salt

1 teaspoon freshly cracked black pepper

1 teaspoon Creole spice blend

2 tablespoons no-sugar-added ketchup

DIRECTIONS

1. Preheat oven to 425°F.

2. In a 9 × 9-inch microwave-safe dish, microwave jicama fries 5
   minutes on high. Cool before handling.

3. In the same dish, brush jicama evenly with olive oil. Sprinkle with Parmesan, salt, black pepper, and creole spices.

4. Spread jicama in one layer, fries not touching, onto a parchment-paper-lined cookie sheet.

5. Bake 35–40 minutes (carefully flipping halfway through baking cycle) until desired level of crispiness is achieved.

6. Serve immediately with no-sugar-added ketchup for dipping.

Pecan-Crusted Chicken Strips

Yield: 6 servings 〉 Prep time: 10 minutes 〉 Cook time: 30–40 minutes 〉
2 net carbs/serving

There are many ways to "bread" chicken on DIRTY, LAZY, KETO, but my favorite is to use crushed pecans. Chicken strips in this recipe taste sweet and salty at the same time—that's my favorite combination! Additionally, I LOVE to crush the pecans. I fill a thick ziplock freezer bag with pecan nuts, then pound them to death using a cast-iron pan. Something about all that smashing is super entertaining and gets all of my stress out.

INGREDIENTS

1½ cups finely crushed pecans

6 packets zero net carbs sweetener, divided

¼ teaspoon salt, divided

2½ pounds of boneless, skinless chicken breasts, cut into 2-inch strips

½ cup (full-fat) mayonnaise

2 tablespoons sugar-free barbecue sauce

DIRECTIONS

Preheat oven to 425°F.

1. In a small baking dish, stir pecans with 5 packets of sweetener and ⅛ teaspoon salt.

2. In a separate dish, coat chicken strips with mayonnaise. Then press each strip firmly into pecan mixture, coating both sides of chicken.

3. Place pecan-covered chicken strips—not touching—on a nonstick wire rack on top of a large, lined baking sheet (for easy cleanup).

4. Cook 10–15 minutes. Turn chicken over gently and bake an additional 10–15 minutes.

5. Sprinkle with remaining sweetener and salt. Serve immediately with sugar-free barbecue sauce for dipping.

A Little Bit? Or Nothing at All?

Our personality types strongly influence our eating behaviors. If you know yourself well, it's easy to tap into your predispositions for help with weight loss. For example, the most powerful thing I learned during my weight-loss journey was that I would rather give up something altogether versus struggling (and failing) with portion control. Instead of torturing myself, I happily eliminated eating popcorn instead of learning to eat "just a little bit" (which is NOT possible, in my opinion). Gretchen Rubin recently put a name to what I discovered to be true so many years ago when I changed my eating habits. In her 2015 book *Better Than Before*, she calls out personality types: "Abstainer" and "Moderator." I am a classic abstainer. I would rather stop eating a food than negotiate the amount to eat.

For my entire life, I felt guilty about not being able to enjoy certain foods in moderation. I could never have "just one" thin mint cookie. Instead, I'd eat the entire sleeve. I felt terrible about my inability to maintain any sense of portion control. What was wrong with me? Why did I lack so much self-control? I carried so much shame around inside. Feelings of guilt gnawed at my self-esteem. I felt like a hopeless failure.

Ironically, once I decided to completely stop trying to moderate eating portions of high-carb foods, *I set myself free*. This freedom is the backbone of DIRTY, LAZY, KETO. By avoiding these foods completely, I instantly became more successful at losing weight *and felt happier*. It's not that being an abstainer was better than being a moderator, I came to realize; this method just worked better for me. Applying this strategy to my dieting was an unexpected breakthrough. I can now sit at a Mexican restaurant and be 100 percent comfortable choosing *NOT* to eat a single tortilla chip from the basket. But if I tried to eat a handful? For me, tasting even one chip would feel like punishment. It would set off my craving to eat the entire basket of chips, and unlimited refills! By leaning into your idiosyncrasies like this, you, too, can better manage the outcome.

The keto way of eating, with its many restrictions, appeals to abstainers like me. We struggle with portion control, and for us, it's easier to completely eliminate entire categories of foods. Bread, pasta, or rice? *No thanks*. Once I stopped eating these foods, I no longer wanted them. These options are literally "off the table," and I feel so much relief.

Rejecting breads (and other starches like rice and pasta) attract a lot of criticism to the keto way of eating. Some argue that categorically cutting out a food group is even dangerous. I've been told I will likely suffer malnutrition because I'm not eating whole grains. *Really? I couldn't disagree more.* Completely avoiding foods like popcorn, crackers, or chips is easier for me. Why do people insist that "everything in moderation" should be a unilateral golden rule? That doesn't work for me. Would you tell an alcoholic to drink small sips of wine? Or demand a former smoker learn to take "just a few puffs"? *I didn't think so.* As a carboholic, I'm no different. Please don't insist I learn to eat quinoa in moderation; respect my decision, and *back the f*#k off!*

#BreakTheRules

These little tricks have helped me to lose more than half of my body weight. They work with, not against, my personality type. I am celebrating, not fighting, my preferences, don't you see?

The most powerful person you can become on this journey is yourself.

By becoming your own advocate, critical comments about what you *should or should not be eating* will roll off your back. Embrace who you are and stop feeling guilty. If you can enjoy a bite of every dish at Thanksgiving dinner and not go "off the rails," then more power to you! But when I tell you that won't work for me, respect my "all or nothing" approach to be just as effective.

4

OH, I CAN'T BECAUSE . . .

Myths, Excuses, and Loopholes—
A Self-Fulfilling Prophecy

Let's tackle common myths and excuses. There shouldn't be any surprises on your DIRTY, LAZY, KETO journey! You will leave here well-equipped to avoid potential land mines. I can already predict what they will be, so I will hand you a detailed road map to follow. Before we get to the nitty-gritty, however, we need to remove the biggest obstacle standing in your path: YOU! You will be quite creative in trying to take yourself on detours, I expect. I anticipate you'll come up with a litany of convincing arguments for why you should quit or cheat. Your excuses will be worthy of an Oscar! Let's address them one at a time.

"I'm Starting Monday"

Starting DIRTY, LAZY, KETO is *not* a court date to dread. There is no need to be nervous, or worse, go off on a binge.

You don't need to eat all the chips and cookies in your house before turning yourself into carb rehab, okay? Putting off a lifestyle change until "Monday" is dangerous because *Monday might never come.* You can always find a seemingly legitimate excuse to postpone getting started. (We can be very convincing when lying to ourselves.) The irony of making excuses, though, is that these justifications *actually make us happy.* By adopting a "believable" defense, we get what we want: *a way out.* Making excuses is a self-fulfilling prophecy.

There is no need to apologize. I know you are afraid. It's unsettling to think about a life without Pepsi (or your favorite foods and drinks). I get it. I'm sure you're worried about feeling deprived, and maybe you're even resentful about having to make a change. Dieting *sucks*, right? Nobody wants to say goodbye to the foods that have been a comfort for so long. It's like breaking up with a hot boyfriend. (Who does that?) I imagine there is a swirl of emotions going on inside of you right now; I know this because I felt overwhelmed, too. I felt anxious, apprehensive, unconvinced, and angry—all at once!

Avoiding the starting line, though, never helped anyone. Waiting "until Monday" (*which can also sound like "I'll start after the holidays" or "I'll start in January" and so on*) isn't the answer. We are going to face this change now—but together—okay? Be brave and take baby steps forward. You can even keep the empty Pepsi can in your hand.

What to Expect—Detoxing and
Sugar Withdrawal

When you stop mainlining carbohydrates, the sugar train comes to a crashing halt. Expect a transition period as your body adjusts. If you were like me and enjoyed *hundreds, if not a thousand,* carbs per day, your body was used to that "feel-good" glucose pumping nonstop. When you go "cold turkey" and switch from glucose to fat for fuel, your body will likely retaliate. At first, expect it to put up a fight. This backlash—feeling achy, tired, and cranky—happens because you are physically "detoxing." Give your body a chance to breathe. Learn to trust your new fuel source—fat. You might even want to "give yourself a break" from working out (if that's something you do) while your body adjusts. Everyone reacts differently. Most people bounce back within a few days.

Claiming they have contacted the "keto flu" is the number-one reason people quit the keto diet.

During the transition period, you might notice how your energy levels change. New patterns will emerge while you become fat-adapted. There will be times in your day when you *surprisingly* feel tired. This is normal. Your body is saying, "*Hey!* What's happening?"

I definitely experienced this. I was used to eating carbs

whenever I felt tired. Chips, cookies, or even dry cereal were my favorite "pick-me-ups." When I stopped eating those foods, I had to fight the urge to try to "fix" feelings of fatigue. Don't laugh, but I needed to learn *how to rest*. Taking a break is a normal part of the day. It doesn't need to be corrected with sugary coffee drinks or high-carb snacks (*which we know just makes it worse in the long run*).

Instead of reaching for carbs, trust the process. Fat adaptation is happening! In the meanwhile, practice other ways to rejuvenate yourself. Get more sleep at night, take an afternoon siesta, or schedule a meditation break in lieu of high-carb snacking. Refresh your energy levels by going outside. Sunshine and a brisk walk work wonders. Soon your body will transition to being fueled by fat instead of carbohydrates, and your energy levels will rebound to all-time highs. Since I started DIRTY, LAZY, KETO, I find myself with more energy than both of my young kids have—*combined!* Have faith, my friend. Power through.

As you wait for ketosis to set in, especially in the beginning, expect to feel predictable symptoms of sugar withdrawal. These symptoms are *not dangerous,* just uncomfortable. It's possible you might experience:

- Severe food cravings
- Moodiness
- Depression
- Anxiety
- Changes with sleep
- Foggy thinking
- Tiredness

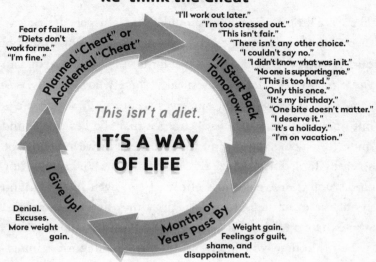

Re-think the Cheat

Planned "Cheat" or Accidental "Cheat"

"I'll work out later."
"I'm too stressed out."
"This isn't fair."
"There isn't any other choice."
"I couldn't say no."
"I didn't know what was in it."
"No one is supporting me."
"This is too hard."
"Only this once."
"It's my birthday."
"One bite doesn't matter."
"I deserve it."
"It's a holiday."
"I'm on vacation."

I'll Start Back Tomorrow...

Fear of failure.
"Diets don't work for me."
"I'm fine."

This isn't a diet.
IT'S A WAY OF LIFE

I Give Up!

Denial. Excuses. More weight gain.

Months or Years Pass By

Weight gain. Feelings of guilt, shame, and disappointment.

Going through sugar withdrawal is not fun. Sugar is as addictive as nicotine! This is another reason why "cheat meals" aren't recommended. Why would you want to put yourself through sugar withdrawal more than you have to? It feels terrible. *Starting DIRTY, LAZY, KETO once is a lot easier than starting over and over, again and again.*

Are you serious about sustainable, long-term weight loss? Or is DIRTY, LAZY, KETO temporary for you? I hope you are committed to making permanent improvements toward living a better life. Cheat meals or cheat days wreak havoc on your weight loss. Eating sugar will confuse your metabolism and derail your confidence. There is a physical and emotional momentum to your weight loss, and I urge you to reconsider any plans to backtrack.

Lies We Tell Ourselves

There is a little devil on your shoulder that whispers destructive theories about why you *can't* lose weight and *why* you should quit. If you tune in, it will even offer up tips on how you can *game the system*. Label this sneaky voice what it really is— *sabotage!* The lies we tell ourselves seem totally legitimate— but only on the surface level. I agree that the lies can sound quite convincing. I urge you to dig deeper, however. Don't be so easily fooled. Recognize the *idiocy* of your "old self" trying to disrupt your weight-loss efforts. I can even forewarn you about the exact lies you will hear, as they are so common. I wrote them all down for you so they are easier to spot.

Self-sabotage will likely fall into two categories: **imaginary obstacles** we think prevent us from losing weight, and **empty justifications** that try to explain "cheating." If I missed one example, be sure to add it to the list. Prepare to giggle or empathize. Even the outrageous alibis remind me of something close to something I've said or thought.

Starting a new way of eating can be daunting. It's like having to make a speech in front of thousands of people—*but naked!* You feel exposed. Instinctually, you try to flee. When we are in precarious positions, all of us look for trapdoors to escape through. We want OUT! Starting a new way of eating is no different. I have heard so many creative excuses. People make up imaginary obstacles *to rationalize why they can't even start.*

Just because you haven't fallen through one of these trapdoors doesn't mean the coast is clear. In addition to justifying

FACEBOOK SHOUT-OUTS

I Can't! Real or Imaginary Obstacles: Stories from the DLK Support Group

"Can I still 'do keto' if I live in a hotel? I don't have a fridge or a gall bladder, either. Can I do this for like forty dollars a month? My husband won't eat these weird foods. Oh, and I have a colostomy bag. Does that matter?" —Unidentified for privacy

"I was doing so well with DLK until my summer trip. I told myself I deserved to eat whatever I wanted. I planned to start again once I got back, but that was six months ago and I still haven't started. I feel so depressed." —Terry

"I'm so tired of seeing the posts that say 'It's okay to cheat because it's the holidays.' Don't they realize it's not worth it? I don't want to end up back on diabetes medicine because of Thanksgiving dinner. My health is worth so much more than a bowl of sweet potatoes." —Randy

"I've struggled with my weight my whole life, so waiting a few more months won't hurt me. I'll start keto again after the holidays. Enjoying a non-keto Christmas doesn't make me less of a person. I want to cook with my mom and be happy." —Sabrina

"Help! I just started. Everything is new and I'm stressed out. I have a business meeting next week, so I'll be traveling. Should I ship food to my hotel or just start over once I get back?" —Maria

"My culture celebrates everything with food. I'm not making excuses or anything, but food is always at the center of our family gatherings. I might be able to eat keto foods during the week, but for family events I have to eat what my family makes." —Anu

"I plan to lose weight with keto but take a break when I have my vacation next month. I want to have fun! I'm celebrating my birthday on the trip." —Karen

why we *can't start* a diet, we often find ways to convince ourselves why we should take *a well-deserved break* from healthy eating. Excuses for going "off the rails" can be so creative! I know you'll identify with quite a few.

Do any of these excuses sound familiar?

Imaginary Obstacles—Trapdoors

- Keto is too expensive.
- My husband/wife/partner won't support me.
- I can't lose weight because of menopause.
- I can't lose weight because of thyroid issues.
- Keto foods aren't available where I live.
- My body is just built this way.
- I don't have time.

- I don't eat avocados.
- I'm allergic to eggs.
- I don't like vegetables.
- I hate eggs.
- My family won't give up junk food.
- I don't have a gallbladder, so I can't do this.
- This way of eating will cause high cholesterol.
- In many cultures, being overweight is beautiful.
- I'm too old.
- I don't have any healthy options.
- I'm a vegetarian.
- I shouldn't have to eliminate food groups; it's not natural.
- I'm fine just the way I am. I don't need to lose weight.
- This food is part of my family's tradition.
- I don't see any other choice here.
- I'm vegan.
- Rice is part of my culture.
- Pasta is part of my culture.
- Genetics prevent me from losing weight.
- I'm going on vacation soon.
- I'm too stressed out. It's not a good time.
- I don't want to lose my curves.
- I'm not at my house right now.
- I travel too much.
- I could never fast.
- But I'm going on a cruise!
- I can't control . . .
- This isn't fair. I want to eat like everyone else.

Cheating vs. Intentional Eating

There is a distinction between "cheating" on a diet versus making a conscious choice to enjoy a taboo food. Cheating is not something you feel proud of. Feelings of shame, disgust, and disappointment surface when cheating. How you rationalize your choice doesn't matter—*but how you feel afterward does*. Are you *proud* of your choice or *ashamed*? Would you *do it again* or are you *full of regret*? This postmortem distinction determines how likely you are to succeed at weight loss.

The Rationalization of "Cheating"

- I deserve this.
- YOLO—You only live once.
- Holidays don't count.
- It's my birthday (or another holiday).
- I've had a bad day.
- I'll go to the gym later to burn this off.
- I deserve a treat.
- There is nothing else I can eat.
- I'm too busy to deal with this today.
- I need a break once in a while.
- I'll start tomorrow.
- Having a cheat meal/day will help me stay on track with the diet later.
- I'll just have a little bit.
- It's a buffet; I need to get my money's worth.
- This holiday wouldn't be special without eating this.

- I just worked out, so I can eat this.
- I'll start again tomorrow.
- It's free!
- I don't want to ask for special treatment.
- I can't waste food.
- I don't have a kitchen.
- One bite doesn't matter.
- I'll start again Monday.
- I'm carb cycling.
- I don't want to hurt the feelings of my hostess.
- A cheat meal will break my weight-loss stall.
- This is a celebration.
- This is too overwhelming.
- This doesn't count.

None of these justifications for cheating make sense. Be honest with yourself! **A cheat meal might taste good *in the moment*, but you might feel embarrassed and regretful once it's over.** Don't get mad, as you know that I am right! There is not one single argument you can make to convince me otherwise. Trying to rationalize this behavior, like "*I deserve it,*" makes no sense. **You deserve better.**

Eating high-sugar, high-carb junk food is not a reward.

Sugar is an addictive poison; let's be honest with ourselves. There are a lot of people in the world that can have a "little bit" of candy or enjoy dessert "once in a while," but *I know I'm not one of those people*. I wouldn't be in this situation if that were true. I've eaten enough popcorn, candy, and chips to last me a lifetime—I don't need another bite to be happy. Once I admitted this truth to myself, the faster I was able to lose weight and confidently keep it off. I had to *stop* playing games and step up to the plate.

What about you? Do you need to "check yourself" against making false excuses?

Anti–cheat mantra: "Eating junk food will not make me feel better about myself."

Note that "I didn't have a choice" also doesn't work. A cheat meal still counts as a cheat meal *even if you didn't plan for it to happen*. You can't blame circumstances for what you eat. No matter if you are at a restaurant, a relative's house, or a work meeting, **you are responsible for your choices.** Do your research. Speak up. Plan ahead. *No excuses.*

What is more important to you—eating these "cheat meals" or being at a healthy weight? I'm going to tell you the truth right now: you can't have both.

Let's have a real conversation. It's hard to see the forest through the trees at this point, I understand. But if you have faith, I absolutely promise you **there is a better life just waiting for you.**

Being consistent with your choices absolutely matters. Staying "on track" with every single thing you put in your mouth—it counts. **Every bite, every meal MATTERS!** Stop lying to yourself and thinking otherwise. It's not even about the food, my friend. *That's* the real secret here. When you consistently make choices that you are proud of, *you are actually honoring and loving yourself.* Every decision you make builds upon the last. Healthy choices, one after another *after another* build your self-esteem and self-confidence. In other words, when you say NO to a cheat meal, you are actually saying, "I AM WORTHY OF A BETTER LIFE!" **This is self-love, people, not punishment.**

FACEBOOK SHOUT-OUT

On and Off the Carb Merry-Go-Round

Story from the DLK Support Group

"Why do I keep doing this to myself? I lose a little bit then start binging on carbs. Afterward, I feel terrible, both physically because my tummy hurts, but also mentally. I beat myself up over falling off a plan that I know works. Why do I keep rewarding (and punishing) myself with food? I hit a short-term goal, then eat a whole cake because I think somehow 'I deserve it.'" —Sarah

Making steady, healthy choices is how to keep the weight off forever. With improved self-esteem, you are capable of anything. That is the goal, right? I want to give you a peak behind the curtain.

There is an existence waiting for you that is more glorious than you may have ever imagined.

There is a life on the flip side of obesity that doesn't leave you feeling sweaty all the time, and that lets you walk up the stairs without huffing and puffing. You'll be able to play on the floor with your grandkids, ride roller coasters, and *run* through the airport to catch a flight. You will have no swelling or headaches and not need medication. Clothes will actually fit. When your loved ones will hug you, their arms will wrap *all the way around*. And I'm just getting started. . . .

The Mythical "Keto Flu"

I want to remove all potential barriers that could affect your success. Other than cheating, the biggest problem beginners face is dehydration. I describe the keto flu as mythical because it's 100 percent preventable. When you lose weight, you pee a lot! You have to counteract this by increasing water and electrolytes in your system, or you risk feeling like garbage.

Symptoms of the mythical "keto flu" can range from mild to severe:

- Heart palpitations or racing heart
- Fatigue
- Dizziness or shakiness
- Headaches or migraines
- Leg cramps or other muscle cramps (especially at night)
- Constipation or a feeling of uncomfortable bloating
- Nausea or vomiting
- Fever

- Overheating or heatstroke due to lack of sweating
- Lack of urination
- Kidney failure
- Seizure
- Coma
- Death

In addition to experiencing changes in your energy levels, when you are losing weight, you also change your body's composition of water weight. While I never personally experienced any serious dehydration problems, I want to forewarn you of the possible consequences if you don't take this section seriously. Mild dehydration can be quickly cured with simple nutritional intervention. Choosing not to follow this route puts you at risk for further complications requiring urgent medical help.

Avoiding the "keto flu" sounds really complicated, but it's actually quite simple: *drink water*! Anticipate your body's increased need for fluids by dramatically increasing your consumption of uncaffeinated drinks.

To prevent dehydration, your body needs additional water and electrolytes. Electrolytes will prevent you from feeling tired and experiencing the mythical "keto flu." Without getting all "scientific" (yup, that word again), I want to give you a quick rundown. Electrolytes are minerals such as sodium, potassium, calcium, and magnesium; they balance the amount of water in your body to help your cells function properly by removing waste products. Do you need to know any of the specifics? *Nope.* You do, however, need to take personal responsibility for increasing electrolytes. Whether or not you experience "keto flu" symptoms is entirely up to you.

How to Boost Electrolytes

- Consume sports drinks that include electrolytes (examples: sugar-free Powerade, Gatorade Zero, Propel, or Smartwater).
- Drink bone broth.
- Sip pickle juice.
- Supplement your water with electrolyte tablets.
- Eat foods rich in *potassium* (nuts, salmon, avocado, leafy green veggies, and mushrooms).
- Eat foods rich in *calcium* (dairy foods like yogurt or cheese, leafy green vegetables, broccoli, fish, almond or coconut milk, canned salmon, shrimp, and peanuts).
- Choose uncaffeinated beverages, such as water, water, and more water.
- Drink oral electrolyte solutions (under advisement of your doctor).

Fasting? But I Like to EAT!

In addition to worrying about contracting the mythical "keto flu," many beginners worry that they have to starve themselves to lose weight. Folks falsely *assume* DIRTY, LAZY, KETO requires fasting. Fasting might have gained mainstream popularity recently, but it's definitely not required for weight loss.

Let's bust this myth wide open: feeling "hangry" is NOT what this is all about! In fact, I recommend the opposite. *Eat!*

#BreakTheRules

I recently went skiing for the first time in twenty years. After losing 140 pounds on DIRTY, LAZY, KETO, I'm finally slim enough that I won't topple over like a wobbly Weeble with two sticks attached to my feet. Aside from my fears about getting on and off the ski lift, I had serious food anxiety about being away from my refrigerator for several hours. I tend to snack a lot, and *not necessarily because I'm hungry*. My snacking might just be a habit, but I also think it's a deeper issue. I have an irrational fear that if I become too hungry, I will lose all self-control and start chowing down on carbolicious treats and gain all of my weight back.

When I hear about people *intentionally* not eating for hours (or days) on end—fasting—I am honestly mystified. How is that possible? And perhaps the more important question: WHY WOULD ANYONE DO THAT if he or she doesn't have to? Before you pick up the phone to call the keto hotline and report me, let me take a pause. If fasting or intermittent fasting is working for you and you find it helpful, let me give you a high five! If it's not, though, or you have anxiety about how often you eat like I do, I want to take a minute and break this down.

Current research shows enormous benefits to fasting. I might be stating the obvious here, but eating less (or not at all) tends to promote weight loss. I get that. Insulin and glucose levels plummet with a lack of food in the body. Weight loss, in turn, reduces the chance of developing diabetes, decreases inflammation, and promotes overall good health. *Well, duh!*

Fasting means you don't eat for a planned amount of time. It seems like a contest on social media lately to see who can fast the longest. Why is this a competition? I'm disturbed by all this bragging. If you couldn't tell anyone about your fast, would you still do it? Aside from legitimate *religious* motivations, why would someone choose to fast? I've heard about the "sixth gear" or mental clarity that people can experience during a fast, but I don't know if I believe it. Mind you, I haven't tried fasting, so I am speaking from total ignorance here, but it sounds horrible. There is probably a technical explanation out there about how fasting resets the body's thermostat and reboots metabolism (Dr. Fung, in his 2016 book *The Obesity Code,* explains this nicely), but is that the REAL reason people fast?

On the surface, fasting seems to be an exercise of self-discipline. People who normally overeat might feel a sense of power when that bad habit is interrupted. I totally understand the desire to stop undesirable behaviors, I do. My ears perk up, however, when I hear people plan a fast as punishment for eating a "cheat" meal. I worry about pendulum-style eating. It seems out of control.

Could fasting be used more positively? Perhaps fasting is not about punishing oneself, but, instead, an opportunity to stop obsessing over food. My judgmental eyes were recently opened with compassion when a friend sheepishly admitted that fasting gives her a feeling of relief. Because she stresses so much about her food choices, a planned fast feels like a vacation from her constant food worries. By hearing her perspective, I realized that we all have a unique path to follow with weight loss. There is no one-size-fits-all approach that is right for everyone. Only you can decide if a planned fast will help or hurt you on your weight-loss journey.

If you're like me and have suffered from obesity most of your life, you may not even know what a hunger pain feels like. I've avoided actual feelings of hunger by eating a constant supply of carbohydrates for decades. I understand that fasting might help some people, but using it to spur weight loss does not appeal to me. I like food too much to take any kind of extended break. I want to feel happy, not "HANGRY." Call me cuckoo, but I'm afraid of feeling hunger pains. That's why I love DIRTY, LAZY, KETO.

What About *Intermittent* Fasting—Is That Different from Fasting?

While fasting means NOT eating for an extended period of time, intermittent fasting (or IF) is a shorter cycle of mini-fasting, usually measured in *hours,* not *days.* There are many variations of IF, like not eating for a set schedule of hours (or within a pattern of days), but all have the same notion: NO FOOD. "Intermittent fasting" is a trendy phrase describing something very simple—not eating. Skipping breakfast or not eating after dinner helps some folks reduce their daily caloric intake. Many people utilize the IF strategy to prevent mindless eating in front of the TV, or to block themselves from eating meals only because "it's time" (even though they aren't even hungry). I completely endorse the IF concept, but I do chuckle when everyone makes a big deal of it by calling this strategy such an important-sounding, scientific-sounding phrase. Instead of calling this intermittent fasting, how about we just say DON'T EAT UNLESS YOU'RE ACTUALLY HUNGRY?

Intermittent fasting is getting a lot of airtime lately in the media. Experts love to glom on to a new idea that could "save the world" from obesity. They claim that fasting (intermittent or otherwise) can improve metabolism, decrease insulin resistance, and help you lose stubborn belly fat. Who am I to argue with such a miraculous discovery?

You might wonder if I incorporated any kind of fasting into my own personal weight-loss experience. Unintentionally, I discovered how an evening "mini-fast" helped me avoid dark hours of binge-eating in front of the television. I'm usually not even hungry at night; the snacking was just a bad habit. I learned to reprogram my inner clock by "closing the kitchen" after cleaning up from dinner. It was as simple as that. When I made this "rule" for myself about not eating in the evenings, it wasn't motivated by official research about resetting my metabolism, I was just trying to stop my Olympic-level snacking. You will have to see what works best for your lifestyle.

Fasting or IF isn't a requirement of DIRTY, LAZY, KETO. Sometimes, these hard-and-fast "rules" can backfire. Telling an overweight person that he or she absolutely MUST "stop eating" at a certain time sounds a lot like the shaming, calorie-restrictive diets that many of us grew up with. Sometimes when we are told we can't do something, the rebel inside of us immediately wants to do the opposite. **If committing to a fast or IF would cause you more harm than good, then don't do it. You know yourself best!**

When following any set of strict rules, as humans we are bound to slip up. And we all know that dieters don't forgive themselves very easily!

In the past, when I screwed up on a "diet," I immediately felt regretful and embarrassed. I would become so angry at myself! Did I forgive myself and move on? Are you kidding me? *Absolutely not!* I would blame myself for being such a fool and feel ashamed for making such an obvious mistake. My mind would race and the negative self-talk would start. My unforgiving thoughts were *horrible*—self-deprecating and downright mean. It didn't just stop there, though. My thoughts would spiral, becoming louder and more frequent until they became . . . *beliefs*.

I'm damn certain you can identify with what I just said. I'm crying now just reading my words over and over again. The devastating path of obesity is like a tornado, with guilt and shame as the eye of the storm. You have to get out of its path. **Be cautious. Protect yourself.** Recognize what self-sabotage talk sounds like so you can change direction.

Self-Sabotage Talk

- I can't do this.
- This is too hard.
- I'm not strong enough.
- I don't have willpower.
- Forget it. I'm done.

Negative self-talk serves no purpose. It derails confidence and erodes self-esteem. Guilt escalates to shame, and before you know it, reverting to old self-destructive behaviors seems plausible.

Yes, You Can

Have we knocked down all of your excuses? "Oh, I can't because . . ." should no longer exist in your vocabulary. There is nothing stopping you, my friend, *but you*. Get out of your own way! Let's do this already.

5

HAVING A BIG-SCREEN TV BUT NOT A GYM MEMBERSHIP

Your Environment Makes or Breaks You

It's no surprise that most, if not all, of the contestants from *The Biggest Loser* television show return home only to eventually regain the weight they worked so hard to lose. On the surface, the reasons they fail might seem obvious to everyone watching at home. The celebrity trainers have moved on, the cameras are turned off, and professional chefs stopped preparing customized meals long ago. But is the reason contestants regain weight that simple? Perhaps the more subtle problem has nothing at all to do with the television show. I believe contestants fail because of the toxic influences waiting for them at home.

If you are now overweight, then your current environment supports an unhealthy lifestyle. There is no judgment here—just a reality check. In fact, should you try to change your weight, I'm betting your environment will fight back and try to stop you. Like any organism, your household will do whatever it takes to try to maintain homeostasis. Is this tendency conducive to weight change? Not at all!

Look around your living room and kitchen and tell me what you see. Are you surrounded by a big-screen television, oversized couch, and a pantry stocked with high-carb, packaged foods? What do you see when you open your fridge? *Uh-oh!* Even if you aren't eating those sugary foods, they are right in front of you. Let's turn to the garage now. How do you get to work, school, or do errands? Are you driving an

SUV, sharing a ride, or traveling on foot? If your day is spent being mostly sedentary (tempted by available, high-carb snacks), losing weight will likely be challenging.

Before you start making excuses (kids, coworkers, your commute, the weather, etc.), I'm going to ask you to *stop being defensive* and think back to your stated weight-loss goal. Keep your eye on the prize. What changes actually need to happen for you to achieve this? Excuses will stop you from making progress. Real life, with all its challenges and temptations, will have an effect on your ability to lose weight. Losing weight doesn't happen in a vacuum. Will your current environment help or hurt you?

You can't expect the world around you to automatically adapt to your "new" lifestyle. If you don't start *proactively* morphing your environment to support nutrition changes *now,* your weight loss will be at risk. Just like *The Biggest Loser* contestant who rebounded after returning to his home, you, too, are likely to regain weight if your household doesn't evolve with you.

My motivation today is to grab you by both sides of your cheeks and lean in so closely that you can smell the chia seed pudding on my breath. I'm going to be loud and assertive, and I won't pussyfoot around.

What are YOU willing to change?

Let's dissect the world you live in with the hope of finding opportunities to make meaningful changes.

Get Back on Your Feet

The other day my family (led by the family dog) was walking to my son's swim-team practice, a distance away of less than a mile. A neighbor drove by and tooted his horn to say hello.

My young son hid his head and turned to me. "Mom, can I ask you an embarrassing question? Are we poor?"

"Huh?" I was taken aback by this question.

My husband and I both work to keep our household afloat. We have a nice roof over our heads and food on the table. While my kids might sometimes wear secondhand clothing, they have never missed a meal.

"No," I replied, almost horrified. "Why do you ask?"

"Because we walk everywhere," my son replied. "It's embarrassing. Everyone else in my school drives to *every-thing,* and we are always *walking.* Don't we have money for gas?"

At that point, I started to chuckle. While I was trying to instill the value of exercise in my kids, I had somehow crossed a line that confused them. Despite having two cars in the driveway, gassed and ready to go, I've chosen a lifestyle where I walk *as much* and *as often* as possible. Even though I live in the suburbs, there are schools, restaurants, and shops within a mile of our house. Call it "being green" or "the dog needs a walk," but in reality, *I need the exercise!* Apparently, my kids think this is embarrassing. They would prefer to join the anti-environment, minivan brigade instead of walk. *Lesson learned.* Your family might be embarrassed by some of the choices you make "in the name of health." The question is, will you let that stop you?

Maybe your opportunity for improvement isn't just about intentional walks. What happens when you're out doing errands? Consider your current modus operandi. If you drive to the store, think about where you park. Do you circle the parking lot like a vulture trying to park in the spots that are closest? What would happen if you made the conscious decision to *always* park far away, just to add in extra "steps"? Imagine the impact little changes could have on your health. Always taking the stairs, instead of the elevator, makes a big difference in the long run. Could you handle this kind of exercise based on what shoes you wear when leaving the house? Do you put on high heels to toddle around in (sorry, gents), or comfortable shoes with some staying power? There are many ways to get around town, and I encourage you to think about how you can change that. Identify what tweaks you will make to increase your activity level. If it helps to think about saving money or the environment, then go with that! Do whatever it takes to cancel the Uber and hit the pavement wearing tennis shoes. Going to the gym once in a blue moon isn't going to be enough. At this juncture, every aspect of your current sedentary lifestyle is up for examination.

I Wanna Get Away: Vacation, Baby!

The kinds of vacations we choose speak volumes about our health. Do you prefer cruises, RV camping, or heading to the spa? Would you say you are more likely to go on adventure travel, attend a theme park, or lie on a beach? Once you are on vacation, what kind of activities do you enjoy? There are certainly no right or wrong answers here, but your immediate response will shed light upon your current values about exercise. If your vacation plans focus on just eating, and not physical activities, you will run into some problems trying to maintain weight loss. If that strikes a chord with you, and maybe even makes you feel defensive, then I've hit the nail on the head. I can just see your furrowed brow and your head shaking side to side, protectively muttering, "You don't know what you're talking about! I walk all the time on the cruise ship."

Or maybe the opposite point of view: "I'm *not* going to DIET while on vacation! We'll be going out to eat!"

Okay, okay, I get it. You don't have to prove anything to me, you know. But maybe when you're done arguing with the page, you could take a moment and think about this further. Could vacations (and overindulging) be what's preventing you from reaching your weight-loss goal?

When I was pregnant with my son, I remember excitedly yammering to a family member about an upcoming weekend cruise I was taking with my husband and his work friends. It would be my first time being on a boat, and all I could think about was the upcoming all-you-can-eat buffets of delicious foods and available spa treatments. I figured since I was pregnant, I could have whatever I wanted. It was going to be a free-for-all! Additionally, since I was delicately "with child," I figured I had a self-appointed hall pass to avoid all exercise. I planned to eat and rest *without a trace of guilt.*

"Doesn't that sound amazing?" I asked my family member, thinking she would agree.

"Hmm . . ." She shook her head no. "Not really my jam," she replied.

I was genuinely surprised by her answer. Stunned, actually. How could someone feel this way about unlimited food? I pushed back: "Why?"

"That doesn't sound like a good vacation to me," she replied. "I'd come home having gained ten pounds."

Whatever, I remember thinking. *Thin people are so weird.*

My vacation planning still includes food, but not food like before. Instead of obsessing about the Mickey Mouse–shaped ice cream at Disneyland, I'm planning where to buy a theme-park turkey leg. My obsession with food hasn't changed; let's be real! My food choices, priorities, and activity levels, though, have certainly evolved.

I believe a vacation isn't a break from real life; it's an opportunity for me to live my life.

Let me share an example.

I recently took the trip of a lifetime to Paris with my family. Now before you get all wide-eyed and "jelly," let me remind you that my second passion beyond DIRTY, LAZY, KETO is cheap travel. I would love to get off topic and share how I nabbed airplane tickets for $119 (SERIOUSLY), but that will get us way off topic. Maybe it's due to our tight budget, and/or my obsession with food, but my first priority for planning our trip was to meet the challenge of finding DIRTY, LAZY, KETO–type foods while in a foreign country. I chose our hotel *not* because it had the best reviews, but because it was adjacent to local grocery stores. *I think that's hilarious.* In a previous life, I might have made excuses to enjoy this once-in-a-lifetime opportunity by eating croissants at every meal. My current self, however, calls out that enticing voice as the big ole liar I know her to be. *Merci beaucoup!*

The truth is that I have already enjoyed enough bread and desserts to last myself a lifetime. Putting myself into a Parisian *carb-coma* won't make me enjoy my vacation any more. In fact, my experience traveling to France was extraordinary. Fueled on full-fat yogurt, artisanal cheeses, and avocado, I walked at least 25,000 steps a day around Paris. I didn't get out of breath, not even once, tromping around every level of the Louvre in a single day. And just because I could, I *raced* my children to the top of the Arc de Triomphe to see who could arrive first, *running up all 284 steps!* That powerful feeling of accomplishment was rewarded with an amazing panoramic view of Paris, something I never thought I would live to see. Bring on more challenges like that trip, I say! *Activities and adventure* make vacation memorable, *not* eating eclairs.

Now that I can comfortably sit in an airplane seat, I feel unstoppable. I want to travel more now that I feel confident that the in-flight seat belt will easily clasp. Yes, the TSA might find all my DIRTY, LAZY, KETO snacks in my carry-on a bit suspicious, but I will take *whatever steps necessary* to maintain my weight loss.

What Are We Doing Tonight?

Before DIRTY, LAZY, KETO, my idea of a good time was to go out to dinner, see a movie, and then grab some dessert. After a long work week, I felt I earned a treat, and eating fried appetizers and buckets of popcorn followed by an ice cream cone seemed like an appropriate reward. I think back to my "old" Friday-night pattern and see so many red flags. I was pretty much going from one eating situation to the next, all under the guise of "deserving it." Now when I hear my inner thoughts suggesting that I've earned some kind of nefarious treat, I immediately counterattack with a positive, productive message like, *"What you really deserve, my love, is a longer, more beautiful life!"*

Separating entertainment from food didn't happen for me overnight. I had to drag some of my loved ones kicking and screaming while I made conscious changes to my Friday-night routine. I had to leave other friends behind. Change isn't easy, especially when it affects other people, that's for damned sure. I had to think about where my problem areas lay. Instead of spending my weekends watching Netflix, I purposefully chose new hobbies that would get me off the couch. I questioned some of the habits my family had, like always going out for ice cream. I looked for new ways we could spend free time together that didn't involve food. I had to really shake things up!

I've had to *relearn* how to entertain myself. I've created new habits like "kickin' it" in lawn chairs with the neighbors on a Friday night, while our kids jump on a trampoline. (I've been known to jump on it myself every once in a while!) I take a ukulele class with my best friend even though I can only strum a handful of chords. My husband and I travel to run races, some far, some close, to keep us motivated to exercise. Our garage holds bikes, tennis rackets, and other sporting equipment that gets used regularly. I shop at thrift stores, search for cheap travel deals online, and volunteer as a race ambassador.* *I write.* These are all "healthy" new ways for me to relax and entertain myself, *none of which revolve around food.*

"But It's My *Birthday*!"

Aside from the "keto flu," the second most common excuse I hear for "falling off the DLK wagon" is "But it's my birthday." It's a curious thing, really, that people would turn a holiday into a day of deliberate self-sabotage. (*Damn, that was harsh.*) Does one piece of cake matter? For most people, probably not. But for you and I? It really does. Let's be honest here. When you rationalize overeating because "it's my birthday," what does that really mean to you? Let me translate what you are *really saying*: "But it's my birthday" means you plan to go overboard—*big time*! You think you "deserve" to eat and drink with wild abandon—no holds barred, guilt-free overindulgence—because you've turned another year older. This plan ALWAYS seems like a great idea until the next day, the next week (or months later, for many people), when the binge finally stops.

Thin people often have a few bites of dessert all the time,

---

* San Francisco Marathon, Bay to Breakers, Berkeley Half Marathon.

this is true. *I am not that kind of a person.* I wouldn't be in this situation if I could eat "just a few bites of cake," before pushing a plate away. *No siree, Bob!* I haven't sent a plate back half full of a dessert for a waiter to toss into the trash can, since . . . um . . . ever!

FACEBOOK SHOUT-OUTS

It's My Birthday!

Stories from the DLK Support Group

"Carbs and calories don't count on your twenty-first, right?" —Jamie

"Yesterday was my birthday. I got up early to go get my free coffee at Starbucks but then somehow talked myself into cake pops and coffee cake, too. I didn't even want them, but because it was my birthday, I thought somehow I needed a treat." —Carol

"Of course I'm going to have cake and ice cream. It's my birthday!" —Lani

"Happy birthday to me! Instead of a cake this year, I'm going to get new makeup. Maybe I'll get new shoes, too." —Mindy

"Don't laugh, but for my birthday this year I made an appointment for a physical. I can't wait for my doctor to see how much I've lost. This is the best present I ever could have given myself." —Juan

This is a controversial topic, for sure. When I hear someone mention, "But it's my birthday," I feel like an alcoholic is saying, "I can handle just one." *Yup, I just went there.* Food addicts also have trouble controlling their food intake; they can't stop at "just one." True, we can't avoid all food, like an alcoholic eliminates alcohol, so maybe this isn't a fair analogy, but you get the point. Now, before you get all wound up about me ruining your birthday, let me admit to you that I've tried (and FAILED miserably) to justify my overeating, too. *It never works.*

I didn't employ the birthday excuse. Instead, I came up with my own creative opportunity to give myself "permission" to binge-eat: running. (*I bet I surprised you with that one.*) Running long distances burns an insane number of calories, and, not surprisingly, the more you run, the more you "get to eat." I wholeheartedly embraced the belief that simple carbs were the most efficient energy source for athletes. (Plus, let's be real here, they taste GREAT!) My poor body was so confused about the game plan. One day I'd be in ketosis and the next day, carbo-loading for long runs.

During my weight-loss journey, when I became a regular runner, I caught on to the fact that my body needed more calories to powerfully run longer distances. I could "get away with" enjoying forbidden foods like bananas, bagels, and even (*gasp*) donuts before a long run. The more I ran, the more carbs I could eat, and before you know it, I was running for hours, *hours* at a time. *I loved it.*

If I only overate for running *once in a while,* this loophole behavior might have been sustainable. By getting to know me here, however, you might have noticed that I rarely do things in moderation. I tend to go OVERBOARD in just about everything I do, and eating excessive amounts of carbs to run was surprisingly no different. Since more running burned more calories, guess what I did? I signed up for a marathon! I realized that training for the marathon distance would award me with maximum opportunities to eat junk food. The experience was addictive. I could eat carbs before long training runs AND I could binge on carbs *practically guilt-free* for several days leading up to the big event of running 26.2 miles. It was a self-fulfilling prophecy!

Runners even had a "scientific" sounding name for binge-eating—"carbo-loading"!

One marathon turned into two, and before you know it, I was so hooked on carbo-loading that I trained for five marathons within a year. Did I love running? Um, yes, but maybe not that much! But do I love eating donuts? *Apparently, yes!*

After injuring my knee and spending a summer with a physical therapist, I had time to reevaluate my behavior. What was I getting out of the marathon distance? I absolutely loved the feeling of accomplishment I got from earning finish line medals, but hated the way my weight would swing up a good ten to fifteen pounds before the big event. *I felt bloated, guilty, and uncomfortable.* I would plan on stopping, *but oh, those carbs tasted good!* I often joked about how much I ate before a marathon, but inside I felt worried. Overeating carbs like that felt unhealthy and shameful, like the way I used to feel when binge-eating in the past.

Because of my precarious history, I've cut way back on committing to races. I approach upcoming runs with more caution. I've spent the last year "working on this." I want to improve my love/hate relationship with food and to experiment with eating enough slow-burning carbs to boost my running, but not so many that my ass starts to eat my running skirt (*which, sadly, has happened*). I'm a work in progress, and that's okay with me.

The bottom line here is a word of caution about loopholes when "eating." While you may think your birthday, marathon, or other special event is "just one day" to overeat, the effects of overindulging, on your self-esteem and waistline, argue differently. Know yourself and your limitations and **make conscious decisions,** knowing the potential repercussions.

Work It, Baby!

Even our careers can become excuses for weight gain. No matter where you work, there will always be temptation to eat carbolicious snacks. People love to show gratitude and appreciation with food, equating sweets with love. These can be hard to resist! Do you have an evil donut-bringer at your work? *Exactly!* In fact, that's probably me (along with a veggie tray). Sometimes people don't know how to show thanks in any other way. Or they share desserts at work that they themselves can't eat. (Anyone raising your hand?) We've all experienced this food phenomenon. Everyone has a unique relationship with food that probably isn't healthy on some level. Compassion and planned responses are needed to navigate the unpredictable landscape of your food at work.

What part of your work life is in your control? Can you pack a lunch, or do you dine with clients? Are you stuck in meetings with catered food, or do you choose where and when you will eat lunch? It's easy to blame your weight on your work situation, as you may feel powerless to make any changes. I urge you to dig deeper, though. Look at the "payoff" you get from playing the blame game. The consequences are dire—guilt, regret, and possible failure. Don't kid yourself by projecting the responsibility of "eating right" onto someone else; you are letting yourself off the hook. *Rethink the cheat.* Take ownership of your circumstances and initiate change.

These days it's not uncommon for folks to openly articulate their special dietary needs. Whether it's a gluten allergy or low-sodium requirement, it's perfectly acceptable to speak up and ask for what you need. You might be surprised at how your dietary requests spark support from those around you! Of course, there are many ways for you to accomplish your goal. Other than asking the waiter for a keto-friendly menu (which he will definitely NOT have!), think about other creative ways to get your needs met.

How Excuses Make Us Happy

Blame	Payoff
I have no time to pack a lunch.	I get to eat fast food.
There are no groceries in the house.	I must eat out.
Someone brought treats to work.	I'm being polite and grateful by eating this.
I didn't choose the restaurant.	I had no choice but to eat that type of food.
The waiter brought me the French fries even though I ordered a side salad.	I can't waste food.
The event was catered with no options.	I couldn't get another type of food if I tried.
I'm eating with a client.	I can't make him/her feel uncomfortable.
Everyone was having this.	I don't want to cause a scene.
I work long hours and have no time to prep meals.	It's not my fault that I have a demanding job.
I spent the morning caring for children and have no time to prep meals.	Others depend on me. Their needs are more important than mine.

Creative Strategies to Stay on Track at Work

- Plan dinners that include leftovers for work the next day.
- Do the grocery shopping yourself: there is no one to blame if you don't have your favorite foods on hand to pack in your lunch.

- Establish new workplace "rules," like brought-in treats should remain on the bringer's own desk to be shared, not left in the break room.
- Know what to order at fast food restaurants. There are more choices at fast food places than you might realize!*
- Buy in bulk (freezing foods, if necessary) to ensure your favorite treats are always in the kitchen for preparing food to take to work.
- Research restaurants ahead of time by going to their websites or calling ahead.
- Store emergency foods at work.
- Prepare meals for the week ahead of time, like on Sunday.
- Invest in appropriate containers to transport and store food safely.
- Buy prepackaged, healthy "convenience" foods, even if they cost more.
- Practice how to order in restaurants (or assertively return what you didn't order to the kitchen, if need be).
- Start new workplace traditions such as bringing balloons instead of cake, to signify birthdays.
- At work conferences or meetings, notify the caterer that you are diabetic. (They understand this more than keto. I'm sorry if I offend anyone with this suggestion—*but it's very effective!*)

---

* *DIRTY, LAZY, KETO Fast Food Guide: 10 Carbs or Less* by William and Stephanie Laska (Amazon, 2018).

Despite our best intentions, there will certainly be times during work or travel when fast food is the best option. Because I've already done so much research on this topic looking at 35 popular restaurants for the bestseller *DIRTY, LAZY, KETO Fast Food Guide: 10 Carbs or Less*, I will briefly provide menu suggestions to get you started. Let's start with Starbucks since coffee is so popular, and then I'll highlight a few fast food restaurants.

Coffee to Go?

Starbucks menu low-carb coffee ideas that are 10 carbs or less.

Starbucks Drink Sizes: Short 8 fl. oz., Tall 12 fl. oz., Grande 16 fl. oz., Venti 20 fl. oz.

Caffè Americano, 2 pumps sugar-free vanilla syrup, Short, 2 g net carbs

Chai Latte, 2 pumps sugar-free Cinnamon Dolce Syrup, Short, 4 g net carbs

Espresso Macchiato with whole milk, Doppio (1.6 fl. oz.), 3 g net carbs

Iced Coffee, 2 pumps of sugar-free Cinnamon Dolce Syrup, Tall, 1 g net carb

Skinny Mocha, with sugar-free Skinny Mocha Sauce, Short, 10 g net carbs

Vanilla Bean Coconutmilk Latte, Short, 10 g net carbs

For Comparison: Coffee (black, unsweetened), Short, 0 g net carbs

"What Should I Order to Eat?"

McDONALD'S

Scrambled egg,* 1 g net carb

Egg McMuffin (no bread), 2 g net carbs

Artisan Grilled Chicken Sandwich (no bun, or substitute lettuce for bread), 2 g net carbs

Turkey Sausage Scramble Bowl, 2 g net carbs

Quarter Pounder with Cheese (no bun, or substitute lettuce for bread), 5 g net carbs

Cheeseburger (no bun, or substitute lettuce for bread), 5 g net carbs

Bacon Ranch Grilled Chicken Salad (no dressing), 5 g net carbs

Side Salad with Newman's Own Light Balsamic Vinaigrette, 6 g net carbs

Big Mac (no bun, or substitute lettuce for bread), 7 g net carbs

Southwest Grilled Chicken Salad (no dressing, no lime glaze, no tortilla strips), 8 g net carbs

BURGER KING†

Sausage Egg & Cheese (no bread), 1 g net carb

Grilled Chicken Sandwich (no bun), 1 g net carb

Double Cheeseburger (plain, no bun), 1 g net carb

BK Ultimate Breakfast Platter (eggs and sausage only), 2 g net carbs

---

* This is not listed on the public menu, although McDonald's will honor this order. You can even request real eggs!

† Burger King does not serve lettuce wraps instead of buns.

Fully Loaded Croissan'wich (no bread), 3 g net carbs

Whopper with Cheese (no bread, no ketchup, 3 g net carbs

Garden Side Salad with Ken's Ranch Dressing, 4 g net carbs

Ken's Golden Italian Dressing, 4 g net carbs

Garden Salad with Grilled Chicken (no dressing, no croutons), 8 g net carbs

Chicken nuggets (4 piece), 10 g net carbs

TACO BELL

Shredded Chicken Burrito (Spicy Ranch Sauce, no tortilla, no beans, no rice), 2 g net carbs

Grilled Breakfast Burrito (request extra eggs, no potatoes, no tortilla), 4 g net carbs

Grande Scrambler Burrito (request extra eggs, no potatoes, no beans, no tortilla), 6 g net carbs

Fresco Burrito Supreme: steak (no rice, no beans, no tortilla), 6 g net carbs

Power Menu Bowl (request extra chicken, extra cheese, extra lettuce, no beans, no rice), 7 g net carbs

Power Menu Bowl: steak (Creamy Jalapeño Sauce, no beans, no rice), 7 g net carbs

Crunchy Taco, 10 g net carbs

CHIPOTLE

Bowl (chicken, no rice, no beans, lettuce, sour cream, cheese), 3 g net carbs

Bowl (steak, no rice, no beans, lettuce, sour cream, cheese), 3 g net carbs

Salad (double steak, light Tomatillo Green-Chili Salsa, sour cream, cheese, lettuce), 5 g net carbs

Bowl (barbacoa, no rice, no beans, lettuce, Fresh Tomato Salsa, sour cream, cheese, and guacamole), 8 g net carbs

Salad (chicken, no dressing, Tomatillo Red-Chili Salsa, sour cream, cheese, guacamole, lettuce), 8 g net carbs

PANERA BREAD

Roasted Turkey & Avocado BLT (no bread), 2 g net carbs

Toasted Frontega Chicken (no bread), 4 g net carbs

Chipotle Chicken Avocado Melt (no bread), 4 g net carbs

Steak & Arugula Sandwich (no bread), 6 g net carbs

Caesar Salad (half portion), 6 g net carbs

Caesar Salad with Chicken (half portion, no dressing), 6 g net carbs

Toasted Steak & White Cheddar (no bread), 7 g net carbs

Greek Salad (no dressing), 7 g net carbs

Green Goddess Cobb Salad with Chicken (half portion, no dressing), 8 g net carbs

Last (*but not least*): The KITCHEN

You might find it ironic that I saved your kitchen at home for last when talking about setting up your environment for success. What's in the kitchen is critical to your success, true, but I actually believe it's just one piece of the larger weight-loss puzzle.

If you haven't cleaned out your kitchen already, there is no time like the present. Grab a giant bag (or box to give it all away, if you're the guilty type) and get rid of all the high-carb crap that caused you to gain weight in the first place. I'm sure you've heard this before, but if you can't find it in your pantry, you won't be able to eat it. Make space, both literally and figuratively, for healthy eating and the "new you." Pay attention to what's going through your thoughts as you select which foods stay and which go, as there is a high probability that *ludicrous self-sabotage is about to start.*

"Oh, that innocent box of brownie mix toward the back of the pantry? I might need it to bake for an upcoming school event."

LIES! *Lies, lies, lies,* I tell you!

I've spent years of my life "making" cake mixes that never even entered the oven. My afternoon snack as a child came from licking chocolate cake batter off a plastic spatula until the bowl was empty. *I can't be the only one!* Toss those Pillsbury boxes into the trash, my friend. You won't be bringing brownies to a picnic anytime soon.

Some foods aren't worth the risk of keeping in the house. If a box of Triscuits might lead you into temptation, toss those crackers in the trash alongside the candy, syrups, and sweet sauces taking up space in your cabinet and fridge. Just because the food isn't full of sugar doesn't mean it's healthy. Sometimes the starchiest crackers are the worst perpetrators. Did you know that biochemically, Ritz Crackers and Keebler cookies have the same effect once they hit the bloodstream? Just ask any diabetic. Both foods are a no-go on DIRTY, LAZY, KETO.

I'm sure there are a few naysayers out there right now, mumbling under their breath about how I'm killing the environment, wasting food, and punishing the rest of the people who live in my house who don't suffer from my weight problem. You know what? You are 100 percent right on every level. *You. Are. Correct.* Now let's move on.

When I did my keto cleanse, you might be curious about how I decided what to keep and what to let go of. **My rule of thumb was to only keep foods in the house that had 10 or fewer net carbs per serving.** If a food had more than that, I got rid of it. Since I was operating with a lean, budgeted amount of 20–50 grams of net carbs per day, I wanted to spend those carbs wisely. I knew from experience that lower carb foods were *less likely* to lead to sugar cravings and would help me lose weight. Getting rid of tempting foods was my best shot at success. Out of sight, out of mind.

Conduct the Keto Cleanse:
Remove or Relocate Tempting Foods

- Bagels
- Baked goods
- Beans
- Bread
- Candy
- Canned fruit
- Canned soup (check label)

- Cereal
- Chips
- Corn
- Crackers
- Desserts
- Dried fruit
- Flavored alcohol (e.g., Baileys, cotton-candy-flavored vodka—*don't judge*)
- French fries
- Frozen dinners
- Frozen pizza
- Fruit juice
- Granola bars
- Honey
- Ice cream
- Instant noodles
- Mashed potatoes
- Milk
- Mixes for brownies/cake
- Muffins
- Oatmeal
- Pasta
- Popcorn
- Potatoes
- Pretzels
- Rice
- Sauces or salad dressings (with more than 3 carbs per serving)
- Soda (not diet)
- Sugar

- Sugary cocktail mixers
- Sweet wines
- Syrup
- Tortillas
- White flour
- Chocolate *(I tried to sneak this one in last so maybe you wouldn't catch it)*

To prevent any interference, I give you permission to conduct your initial "carb extermination" while you are home *alone* and everyone else is gone to work or school—*anywhere but in your way.* The keto cleanse is not meant to be a group project in which arguments ensue about what defines healthy eating. No one has to know what you are up to! When your family starts complaining about the lack of chips or ice cream in the house, tell them to add it to the shopping list. *Next, throw that list away when no one is looking.* Problem solved, *right?*

I am being a little facetious here when suggesting you don't need to consider other people's needs within your household (*as long as you know that your needs are most important!*). I understand that logistically and financially, you might not be able to remove 100 percent of these foods without dire consequences. I certainly don't want divorce papers filed or a staged teenage rebellion to ensue. I get it! Perhaps there is another approach that is less "extreme low-carb makeover," and a bit more sensitive. Instead of throwing junk food away, could you reorganize your kitchen/pantry space? I'd like to suggest an alternative (though potentially less effective) method for making your low-carb choices more prominent. In both your fridge and pantry, commandeer all of the eye-level shelves for your "safe" foods. Relocate foods you'd like to avoid to a less desirable, more inconvenient location.

#BreakTheRules

From experience, I know that my eyes (not my brain) make most of my food decisions. When DIRTY, LAZY, KETO snacks and meals are at eye level and easy for me to reach, I am more likely to choose those foods—*every single time.* Hypothetically, if I have to drag a chair across the kitchen floor and stand on it to access the cabinet above the fridge, I am *much less likely* to look for snacks in that location. I'm just too lazy! Reorganize your kitchen according to your new priorities, and you will have set yourself up for success.

I remember searching the cabinets for "something sweet" and coming up empty. In my desperation, I gnawed on a baking square of chocolate, which tasted only one notch above eating dirt.

Let's Go Shopping

Once your kitchen is reorganized, it's time to go to the store. Get out there and stock your kitchen with foods to help you lose weight. *No excuses.*

Shop the perimeter of the grocery store (not up and down the aisles). The perimeter of the store is where you will find (what we call lovingly in my house) "REAL FOOD." What is real food, you ask? Real foods don't come in a box; rather, they're grown in soil, raised on a farm, or swim in the ocean. *Eggs, meat, fruit, and vegetables* are examples of real food.

I am providing my grocery shopping list here to get you started, but by no means are you "required" to purchase these recommendations. These are suggestions meant to push you in the right direction, or maybe to reinspire you. This is the current working grocery list I personally use to feed my family. It took *years* to fine-tune the items shared here! I didn't buy all of these items at once. Rather, I chipped away at stocking my kitchen shelves over time. As I discovered new foods that met my "10 net carbs or less" criteria and fit my DIRTY, LAZY, KETO lifestyle, I added them to this master grocery list. Low-carb, high-fat, moderate-protein foods that are *also* high-fiber should earn a gold star. These are the coup de grâce of the DIRTY, LAZY, KETO weight-loss experience and are highly recommended for your shopping cart.

Many surprised DLK followers share that their grocery bill goes down. Replacing packaged junk food (cookies, chips, cereals, crackers, soda) with "real food" saves big money!

What about brands? Unless the item is unique, like Carbquik, for example, I rarely recommend a specific brand. Sure, I have my favorites, like Bob's Red Mill or Quest, but I also like trying new products and catching a good sale! Be sure to check the nutrition label of whatever foods you choose to buy, as brands differ with carb counts even among the same item. For example, I've noticed that almond flour and marinara sauce differ in net carbs according to the manufacturer. Be sure to shop around for the best carb offering.

Grocery Shopping Hacks

- Make shopping a regular routine, like every Monday after work.
- Bring a list.
- Do the shopping yourself, so you can't blame someone else for buying the wrong foods.
- Just because the package says "keto" on it doesn't mean you need it.
- There are no "fancy ingredients" required, just real food.
- Shop the perimeter of the store, where fresh food is restocked often.
- Take shortcuts if necessary. (Try rotisserie chicken, premade kabobs, bagged lettuce, frozen riced cauliflower, etc.)
- Buy more vegetables than you think you need. VEGETABLES ARE A GREAT INVESTMENT IN YOUR HEALTH.

Save Money

- Buy DLK-friendly ingredients over time. Like you would with a good wardrobe, purchase ingredients as you need them, or as a "treat," but not all at once.

- Plan for leftovers. I find that by making a big Crock-Pot full of shredded chicken, for example, I am able to make multiple meals several days in a row.
- Utilize your freezer. Buy in bulk to reduce costs. Watch for sales.
- Avoid costly and unnecessary "keto junk food" purchases, like low-carb ice cream, protein bars, and keto chips. Because I know you are curious, I will include some of these in the grocery list, but by no means am I insisting you must have them! Luxury purchases like sugar-free barbecue sauce or sugar-free coffee syrups are *not a necessity*.
- Challenge yourself to find the best prices by visiting different grocery stores or through buying favorite items in bulk.
- Buy fresh vegetables that are in season, as they are lower in cost, or swap out frozen for fresh.
- Explore ethnic grocery stores for unique spices and fresh ingredients.
- Compare prices to online sources for the best deals.

No matter what your budget is, DIRTY, LAZY, KETO is possible. Do not give up on losing weight because you think you can't afford it.

DIRTY, LAZY, KETO Grocery List

DRINKS

Beer (low-carb), varies per brand, estimated 3–5 g net carbs per 12 fl. oz. serving

Coffee (black), 0 g net carbs per 8 fl. oz. serving

Diet soda, 0–1 g net carbs per 8 fl. oz. serving

Electrolyte water (MiO, Powerade, Smartwater), 0 g net carbs per 8 fl. oz. serving

Energy drinks (sugar-free or low-carb), 0–3 g net carbs per 8 fl. oz. serving

Flavored drink mix packets or squirts, sugar-free, 0–3 g net carbs per ½ packet serving

Hot cocoa mix (note that fat-free hot cocoa mix *has substantially fewer* net carbs than hot cocoa mix with no sugar added!), 4 g net carbs per (8 gram) envelope serving

Juice, diet (sugar-free grape, sugar-free cranberry*), 2 g net carbs per 8 fl. oz. serving

Liquor (unflavored hard alcohol), 0 g net carbs per 1.5 fl. oz. serving

Malt beverages, low-carb (varies per brand), estimated 1–5 g net carbs per 12 fl. oz. serving

Milk (unsweetened, dairy alternative milk: almond, coconut, cashew, flaxseed, hemp, or soy milks), estimated 0–2 g net carbs per 1 cup serving

Mineral water or naturally flavored water (sugar-free), 0 g net carbs per 8 fl. oz. serving

---

* Ocean Spray, diet juice sweetened with Sucralose

Seltzer water (sugar-free), 0 g net carbs per 8 fl. oz. serving

Soda water (sugar-free), 0 g net carbs per 8 fl. oz. serving

Tea (unsweetened, sugar-free: herbal, black, green), 0 g net carbs per 8 fl. oz. serving

Tonic water (sugar-free), 0 g net carbs per 8 fl. oz. serving

Water (flat), 0 g net carbs per 8 fl. oz. serving

Wine (dry), 3–4 g net carbs per 5 fl. oz. serving

DAIRY (ALWAYS CHOOSE FULL-FAT)

Butter, 0 g net carbs per 1 tablespoon serving

American cheese (processed cheese food), 1–2 g net carb per 1 slice (19–21 gram) serving

Asiago cheese, 0 g net carb per 1 oz. serving

Blue cheese, 1 g net carb per 1 oz. serving

Brie cheese, 0 g net carb per 1 oz. serving

Cheddar cheese, 1 g net carb per 1 oz. serving

Cheese (full-fat, block or shredded), 0–1 g net carb per 1 oz. serving

Colby jack cheese, 1 g net carb per 1 oz. serving

Cottage cheese, 4% milk fat, 5 g net carbs per ½ cup serving

Cream cheese, 2–3 g net carbs per 2 tablespoon serving

Eggs, 1 g net carbs per 1 medium egg serving

Feta cheese, 1 g net carb per ¼ cup serving

Ghee, 0 g net carbs per 1 tablespoon serving

Goat cheese, 0 g net carb per 1 oz. serving

Gorgonzola cheese, 1 g net carb per 1 oz. serving

Gouda cheese, 0 g net carb per 1 oz. serving

Gruyere cheese, 0 g net carb per 1 oz. serving

Half-and-half (full-fat), 1 g net carb per 2 tablespoon serving

Heavy whipping cream, 0 g net carbs per 1 tablespoon serving

Ice cream (low-carb*), varies per brand, estimated 0–1 g net carb per ½ cup serving

Milk (unsweetened, dairy alternative milk: almond, coconut, cashew, flaxseed, hemp, or soy milks), 0–2 g net carbs per 1 cup serving

Monterey jack cheese, 0 g net carb per 1 oz. serving

Mozzarella cheese, 1 g net carb per ¼ cup serving

Muenster cheese, 0 g net carb per 1 oz. serving

Parmesan cheese, 1 g net carb per 1 oz. serving

Pepper jack cheese, 0 g net carb per 1 oz. serving

Provolone cheese, 1 g net carb per 1 oz. serving

Ricotta cheese (whole milk), 3 g net carb per ¼ cup serving

Sour cream (full-fat), 1 g net carb per 2 tablespoon serving

String cheese, 1 g net carb per 1 piece (28 gram) serving

Swiss cheese, 0–1 g net carb per 1 oz. serving

Velveeta cheese, 3 g net carb per 1 oz. serving

Whipped heavy cream in can (sugar-free), 0 g net carbs per 2 tablespoon serving

Whipped dairy topping in can (regular), 1 g net carb per 2 tablespoon serving

---

* Popular low-carb brands of ice cream: Enlightened, Halo Top, Rebel

Yogurt (varies per brand), estimated 3–9 g net carbs per
  1 cup serving

MEAT AND SEAFOOD

Bacon (unflavored), 0 g net carbs per 2 cooked slice
  (19 gram) serving

Beef, 0 g net carbs per 3 oz. serving

Chicken, 0 g net carbs per 4 oz. serving

Chorizo (beef, pork, soy), 4–7 g net carbs per 2 oz.
  serving

Deli meat (varies per brand), 0–2 g net carb per 2 oz.
  serving

Duck, 0 g net carbs per 4 oz. serving

Edamame, 3 g net carbs per ½ cup serving

Eggs, 1 g net carbs per 1 medium egg serving

Gyro meat, 5–7 g net carbs per 2 oz. serving

Hot dog (varies per brand), estimated 2 g net carbs per 1
  link (42 gram) serving

Jerky (varies per brand), estimated 3 g net carbs per
  serving

Lamb, 0 g net carbs per 3 oz. serving

Lunch meat (varies per brand), estimated 0–2 g net carbs
  per 2 oz. serving

Meat substitute, formed vegetable protein (varies per
  brand and style: crumbles, nuggets, patty), estimated
  1–15 g net carbs per 3 oz. serving

Pepperoni, 0 g net carbs per 15 slice (28 gram)
  serving

Pork, 0 g net carbs per 3 oz. serving

Rotisserie chicken, 0 g net carbs per 4 oz. serving

Sausage, breakfast (varies per brand), estimated 0–2 g net carbs per 2–3 link serving

Seafood (fish, shellfish, shrimp, lobster),* 0 g net carbs per 3 oz. serving

Spam, 1 g net carb per 2 oz. serving

Tofu, 1–2 g net carbs per 3 oz. (1″ slice) serving

Turkey, 0 g net carbs per 3 oz. serving

PRODUCE†

Alfalfa sprouts, 0 g net carbs per 1 cup serving

Artichoke, 5 g net carbs per ½ cup serving

Arugula, 1 g net carb per 1 cup serving

Asparagus, 2 g net carbs per 1 cup serving

Avocado, 1 g net carbs per ⅓ of a medium (50 gram) avocado serving

Bamboo shoots, 5 g net carbs per 1 cup

Bean sprouts, 4 g net carbs per 1 cup serving

Beans (green, wax, Italian), 2 g net carbs per ½ cup serving

Bell pepper (green), 4 g net carbs per 1 cup serving

Bell pepper (red), 12 g net carbs per 1 cup serving

Bell pepper (yellow), 8 g net carbs per 1 cup serving

Blackberries, 6 g net carbs per 1 cup serving

Blueberries, 18 g net carbs per 1 cup serving

Broccoli (fresh), 4 g net carbs per 1 cup serving

Broccoli (frozen), 2 g net carbs per 1 cup serving

---

* Avoid imitation crab meat, which has added sugar.
† We all know that fresh produce is ideal, but if your budget or geography prevents you from accessing fresh fruits and vegetables, substitute canned or frozen. *No excuses!* I emphasize budget options in my upcoming book, *The DIRTY, LAZY, KETO Dirt Cheap Cookbook* (Simon & Schuster, Fall 2020).

Brussels sprouts (cooked from fresh), 3 g net carbs per ½ cup serving

Cabbage (bok choy), 1 g net carb per 1 cup serving

Cabbage (green, raw), 3 g net carbs per 1½ cup serving

Cauliflower (raw), 3 g net carbs per 1 cup serving

Cauliflower (riced), 2 g net carbs per ½ cup serving

Celery (raw), 1 g net carb per 1 cup serving

Chayote, 4 g net carbs per 1 cup serving

Chicory greens, 0 g net carbs per 1 cup serving

Chinese cabbage, 1 g net carb per 1 cup serving

Coleslaw mix, 3 g net carbs per 1½ cup serving

Collard greens (cooked), 3 g net carbs per 1 cup serving

Cucumber (raw), 2 g net carbs per 1 cup serving

Daikon (oriental radish, raw), 3 g net carbs per 1 cup serving

Edamame, 4 g net carbs per ½ cup serving

Eggplant, 2 g net carbs per 1 cup serving

Endive, 0 g net carb per 1 cup serving

Escarole, 1 g net carb per 1 cup serving

Garlic (fresh), 1 g net carb per 1 clove serving

Ginger, 2 g net carb per 5 slice (1″ in diameter) serving, 1 g net carb per 1 tablespoon ground serving

Green bean (string, raw), 4 g net carbs per 1 cup serving

Green onion (raw), 4 g net carb per 1 cup serving

Greens (collard, cooked), 3 g net carbs per 1 cup serving

Greens (kale, cooked from fresh), 2 g net carbs per ½ cup serving

Heart of palm (canned), 3 g net carb per 1 cup serving

Herbs, fresh (cilantro, parsley, rosemary, thyme), 0 g net carbs per 1 tablespoon serving

Jalapeño (fresh), 1 g net carb per ¼ cup serving

Jicama (raw), 5 g net carbs per 1 cup serving

Kale (cooked), 2 g net carbs per ½ cup serving

Leeks (cooked), 6 g net carbs per ½ cup serving

Lemon (fresh fruit), 4 g net carbs per medium fruit (2⅛" in diameter) serving

Lemon (juice only), 0 g net carb per teaspoon, 1 g net carbs per 1 tablespoon serving, 15 g net carb per 1 cup serving

Lettuce and salad mixes, 1–2 g net carbs per 2 cup serving

Lime (fresh), 5 g net carbs per medium fruit (2⅛" in diameter) serving

Lime (juice only), 0 g net carb per teaspoon, 1 g net carbs per 1 tablespoon serving, 19 g net carb per 1 cup serving

Mushroom (raw), 2 g net carb per 1 cup serving

Mustard greens, 1 g net carb per 1 cup serving

Okra, 4 g net carb per 1 cup serving

Onion (red, yellow, white), 12 g net carbs per 1 cup serving

Pumpkin (fresh), 7 g net carbs per 1 cup cubed serving

Snow peas, 4 g net carbs per 1½ cup serving

Peperoncini (sliced), 0–1 g net carbs per 12 piece (30 gram) serving

Radicchio lettuce, 1 g net carb per 1 cup serving

Radish, 2 g net carbs per 1 cup serving

Raspberries, 7 g net carbs per 1 cup serving

Red onion, 12 g net carbs per 1 cup serving

Rhubarb, 3 g net carbs per 1 cup serving

Romaine lettuce, 1 g net carb per 1 cup serving

Rutabaga (raw), 9 g net carbs per 1 cup serving

Salad greens, 0–1 g net carbs per 2 cup serving

Snap pea, 4 g net carbs per 1½ cup serving

Spinach (raw), 0 g net carb per 1 cup serving

Sprout (alfalfa), 0 g net carbs per 1 cup serving

Squash (spaghetti), 6 g net carbs per 1 cup serving

Starfruit, 3 g net carbs per 1 medium sized fruit (3–5⅛"
long) serving

Strawberries, 8 g net carbs per 1 cup serving

Swiss chard, 2 g net carbs per ½ cup serving

Tomatillo, 1 g net carb per ¼ cup serving

Tomato, 4 g net carbs per 1 medium-sized whole fruit
(123 gram) serving

White onion, 12 g net carbs per 1 cup serving

Yellow onion, 12 g net carbs per 1 cup serving

Zucchini, 3 g net carbs per 1 cup (chopped) serving

Zucchini, 2 g net carbs per 1 cup (sliced) serving

BAKING

Almond flour (super-fine), 3 g net carbs per ¼ cup serving

Almonds, 3 g net carbs per 1 oz. serving

Baking powder, 1 g net carb per 1 teaspoon serving

Baking soda, 0 g net carb per 1 teaspoon serving

Brazil nuts, 1 g net carb per 1 oz. serving

Cacao 100% unsweetened baking chocolate, 1 g net carb
per 2 piece (14 gram) serving

Cacao 85–86% chocolate, 6 g net carbs per 2.5 pieces (30 gram) serving

Cacao 92% chocolate, 6 g net carbs per 3 pieces (34 gram) serving

Cacao powder (cocoa powder) 100% unsweetened, 1 g net carb per 1 tablespoon serving

Chia seeds (black, whole), 3 g net carb per 2½ tablespoon serving

Cocoa roasted almonds, 3 g net carbs per 1 (17.5 gram) packet

Chocolate candy,* varies according to brand, estimated 1–2 g net carb per 2–5 piece serving

Chocolate chips (sugar-free, *sweetened with malitol†*), 8 g net carbs per 1 tablespoon serving

Chocolate chips (sugar-free, *sweetened with stevia‡*), 1 g net carb per 60 chips (14 gram) serving

Chocolate snack bar (Atkins), estimated 2–4 g net carbs per 1 (1.4 oz.) bar

Chocolate syrup, sugar-free, 1 g net carb per 1 tablespoon serving

Chocolate frozen dessert bar§ (sugar-free or no sugar added), varies per brand, estimated 2–6 g net carb per bar serving

Coconut (unsweetened, shredded), 2 g net carbs per 2 tablespoon serving

Coconut flour, 4–5 g net carbs per ¼ cup serving

---

* Russell Stover Assorted Sugar-free Chocolates, Hershey's Sugar-free Chocolate
† Hershey's Kitchens Baking Chips
‡ Lily's Sweets
§ Popular brands of frozen chocolate treats include Breyers Carb Smart, Enlightened, and Popsicle.

Creole seasoning blend, 0 g net carbs per ¼ teaspoon
   serving
Flaxseed (ground), 1 g net carb per 2 tablespoon serving
Flaxseed meal (whole), 2 g net carb per 2½ tablespoon
   serving
Gelatin (sugar-free), 0 g net carb per ½ cup serving
Hazelnuts, 2 g net carbs per 1 oz. serving
Hemp seeds (shelled), 1 g net carbs per 3 tablespoon
   serving
Macadamia nuts, 2 g net carbs per 1 oz. serving
Oil (canola, coconut, grapeseed, olive, peanut, sesame,
   sunflower, safflower, walnut), 0 g net carb per 1
   tablespoon serving
Peanuts (roasted, salted), 3 g net carbs per 1 oz. serving
Pecan nuts (halves), 1 g net carbs per 1 oz. serving
Protein powder* (varies per brand), estimated 1–5 g net
   carbs per 1 scoop (30 gram) serving
Psyllium husk powder, 1 g net carb per 1 teaspoon
   serving
Pumpkin (canned), 6 g net carbs per ½ cup serving
Pumpkin seeds (roasted and salted), 2 g net carbs per
   ¼ cup serving
Seeds (chia, flax, hemp, pumpkin, sesame, sunflower),
   5–11 g net carbs
Sesame seeds (raw), 4 g net carbs per 1 oz. serving
Soy flour, 5 g net carbs per ¼ cup serving
Sugar substitute (Splenda, Swerve, monk fruit, etc.),

---

* Quest brand offers a variety of low net carb protein powders.

0–1 g net carbs per 1 teaspoon (4-gram packet) serving

Sunflower seeds, 4 g net carbs per ¼ cup serving

TVP* (Textured Vegetable Protein), 3 g net carb per ¼ oz. serving

Vanilla (imitation flavoring), 0 g net carb per ⅛ teaspoon serving

Vanilla (pure), 0 g net carbs per ⅛ teaspoon serving

Vital wheat gluten flour, 3 g net carbs per ¼ cup serving

Walnut (halves and pieces), 2 g net carbs per 1 oz. serving

Xanthan gum, 0 g net carbs per 1 tablespoon serving

SAUCES & SPICES

Au jus gravy mix powder, 1 g net carb per ¼ cup prepared gravy serving

Barbecue sauce (sugar-free), 2 g net carbs per 2 tablespoon serving

Black pepper, 1 g net carb per 1 teaspoon serving

Bouillon, 0–1 g net carb per ½ cube or ¼ cup prepared serving

Cinnamon (ground or stick), 0 g net carb per ⅛ teaspoon serving

Curry powder, 0 g net carb per ⅛ teaspoon serving

"Everything but the Bagel" spice *(completely unnecessary, but delicious!)*, 0 g net carb per ¼ teaspoon serving

---

* TVP by Bob's Red Mill

Garlic (powder), 6 g net carb per 1 tablespoon serving, 2 g net carb per 1 teaspoon serving

Hot sauce (varies among brands), estimated 0–1 g net carbs per 1 teaspoon serving

Italian seasoning blend, 0 g net carbs per ¼ teaspoon serving

Ketchup (no-sugar added), 1 g net carbs per 1 tablespoon serving

Marinara sauce* (no sugar added), 4 g net carbs per ½ cup serving

Mayonnaise (full-fat), 0 g net carbs per 1 tablespoon serving

Mustard (yellow, spicy, or dry), 0 g net carbs per 1 teaspoon serving

Pancake syrup (sugar-free), 0 g net carb per ¼ cup serving

Ranch powder mix, 1 g net carb per ½ teaspoon serving

Salad dressing (suggestion: blue cheese, Caesar, creamy Italian, ranch), 1–3 g net carbs per 2 tablespoon serving

Salt, 0 g net carbs per ⅛ teaspoon serving

Soy sauce, 1 g net carb per 1 tablespoon serving

Sriracha sauce, 1 g net carbs per 1 tablespoon serving

Syrup (flavored, sugar-free, for coffee), 0–1 g net carbs per 2 tablespoon serving

Taco powder seasoning, 3 g net carbs per 2 teaspoon serving

---

* Finding low-carb marinara sauces can be a challenge depending on your budget and where you live. Some popular brands include Rao's Homemade or Hunt's Pasta Sauce—*No Sugar Added*.

Turmeric powder, 0 g net carb per ⅛ teaspoon serving

Vinegar (apple cider vinegar, plain white), 0 g net carb per 1 tablespoon serving

Worcestershire sauce, 1 g net carb per 1 teaspoon serving

CANS, BOTTLES, AND JARS

Alfredo sauce, 4 g net carbs per ¼ cup serving

Barbeque sauce (sugar-free), 2 g net carbs per 2 tablespoon serving

Broth (canned), 1 g net carb per 1 cup serving

Chicken (canned), 0 g net carbs per 2 oz. serving

Chiles (green, diced), 6 g net carb per ½ cup serving

Clams (canned), 2–3 g net carbs per 3 oz. can serving

Coconut milk (unsweetened, 12–14% fat), 1 g net carbs per 2.7 fl. oz. or ⅓ cup serving

Crab meat* (real, canned), 2 g net carb per 4.25 oz. can serving

Enchilada sauce (green or red), 4 g net carb per ¼ cup serving

Gravy (turkey, chicken, beef), estimated 3–4 g net carb per ¼ cup serving

Jam, Jelly, and Preserves (sugar-free), 3–5 g net carbs per 1 tablespoon serving

Lemon juice, 0 g net carb per teaspoon, 1 g net carbs per 1 tablespoon serving, 15 g net carb per 1 cup serving

---

* Avoid imitation crab meat, which contains added sugar.

Lime juice, 0 g net carb per teaspoon, 1 g net carbs per 1 tablespoon serving, 19 g net carb per 1 cup serving

Nut butter or no-sugar-added peanut butter, 3–6 g net carbs per 2 tablespoon serving

Olives (black, green), 1 g net carb per 2 (large) olive serving, 1 g net carb per 5 (medium) olive serving

Peanut butter, 6 g net carb per 2 tablespoon serving

Pesto, 1–5 g net carbs per ¼ cup serving

Pickles (dill),* 1–2 g net carbs per ¾ spear (1 oz.) serving

Pumpkin (100% pure, canned), 6–8 g net carbs per ½ cup serving

Salmon (canned), 0 g net carbs per 5 oz. can serving

Sardines (canned in oil), 0 g net carbs per ¼ cup serving

Tuna (canned in oil), 0 g net carb per 2 oz. serving

Vienna sausage, 1 g net carb per ½ can (60 gram) serving

MISC.

Chocolate frozen dessert bar† (sugar-free or no sugar added), varies per brand, estimated 2–6 g net carb per bar serving

Gum (sugar-free), 0 g net carbs per 1 stick serving

Hard candy (sugar-free), varies per brand, estimated 0–1 g net carbs per 4–6 piece serving

Popsicles (sugar-free), varies per brand, estimated 4 g net carb per popsicle serving

Pork rinds (*I don't like these myself, but my husband loves these!*), 0 g net carbs per .5 oz. serving

---

* Avoid sweet and sour pickles (unless sugar-free variety).
† Popular brands of frozen chocolate treats include Breyers Carb Smart, Enlightened, and Popsicle.

Protein bar (Quest), 4 g net carbs per 1 bar (200 gram) serving

Tortillas* (low-carb), 4–6 g net carbs per medium-sized tortilla serving

ONLINE PURCHASE

While most DIRTY, LAZY, KETO ingredients are available at your local grocery store, these last few items are best found online:

Black soy beans† (canned), 1 g net carb per ½ cup serving

Carbquik Baking Mix,‡ 2 g net carbs per ⅓ cup serving

MCT oil, 0 g net carbs per 1 tablespoon serving

Specialty Stores

Does it matter where you buy your groceries? Let me come out ahead and address any reservations you might have: **you don't need to be rich or have access to specialty stores to enjoy the DIRTY, LAZY, KETO way of eating.**

If your family values lead you to shop at a farmers' market for organic, locally grown, responsibly sourced "this and that," more power to you! If you are on my budget, however, and healthy fresh foods start to scare your debit card back into hiding, I've got a plan for you. Drumroll, please . . .

---

* Popular low-carb brands of tortillas include Mission Carb Balance and La Tortilla Factory Low Carb.
† Eden Foods brand.
‡ Carbalose™ baking mix manufactured by Tova Industries.

discount grocery stores! Bargain bliss might be just a block or two away.

Depending on where you live, you might be surprised to discover fresh, frozen, or canned groceries being sold at blockbuster discounts. I have been able to try new foods and recipes for myself and my family without a fear of wasting money. Discount stores sell the same brand names as I find in my local supermarket, but often with a shorter expiration date.

Trust me when I tell you that saving money is an absolute passion of my family. In fact, my husband and I have been compiling all our secrets to include in *The DIRTY, LAZY, KETO Dirt Cheap Cookbook** coming out in the fall of 2020.

Vegetables are available no matter what your budget. Every community has opportunities to save money buying vegetables, whether they're at a Walmart Supercenter or an open-air farmers market. Find a way to get them into your cart. Plant a garden. Join a co-op. Sign up for an online delivery service. If it's important to you, *you'll find a way.*

Final Words of Encouragement

Whether it's parking far away from your destination, packing leftovers to eat at work, or choosing a vacation that encourages activity, every bit of activity in your environment matters. The kitchen is just one piece of the puzzle. Stocking your fridge wisely won't solve all of your problems. Stop blaming

---

* *The DIRTY, LAZY, KETO Dirt Cheap Cookbook* by Stephanie and William Laska (Simon & Schuster, 2020).

the world around you for missteps that you are in control of. Take ownership of your life, at home, at work, and on the road! Instead of listing all the reasons why you can't change, focus on what you can do: **be part of your solution.** Surround every bit of your life with ways to support a "thinner" lifestyle. I promise, your new life is every bit worth the effort.

6

EATING OUR FEELINGS: THEY TASTE DELICIOUS!

Is a Frappuccino Straw an Adult Pacifier? Looking for Comfort in All the Wrong Places

If I only ate when I was hungry, I wouldn't be challenged with weight problems. Instead, I was brought up to celebrate every occasion with food, to snack whenever I felt bored, and to binge-eat to cope with loneliness, boredom, and stress. No matter what emotion I was feeling, it's been programmed in me to pair the feeling with food. No wonder I'm such a mess!

How did this happen? Annual birthday cakes, ice cream cones, and champagne toasts have punctuated celebrations throughout my life. Further, I learned at a young age that eating sweets would physically ease emotional heartache. I've internalized the message that food isn't meant just for nutrition; it also serves up comfort and entertainment. Thanksgiving? Christmas? We are *supposed* to overeat on holidays. Sadly, I hear, "You deserve a break today" on the radio, and

I start driving toward McDonald's *because I deserve a treat.* It's been ingrained in me that I have to soothe myself primarily with food and drinks. Food never lets me down. It's cheap and always available. More important, no matter what I'm feeling, eating food (especially sugar and carbs) makes me feel good (*albeit temporarily*). **Food is a socially acceptable drug that we think will work.**

I once had a friend tell me an intimate food confession that proves this point. On her way home from work, she frequently stopped by a pastry store to buy two dozen assorted donut holes. She would ask for a second, empty bag after paying the tab.

"I would slowly chew each donut hole, one by one, but then spit it out into the second bag," she whispered, disgusted with herself.

She went on, coming clean that before arriving home to her family, she would throw the bag of chewed food out the window from her moving car, removing all evidence *like it never happened.*

That story stuck with me, not because it's kind of gross, but because it was the first time that I ever heard someone *so honestly* talk about his or her warped eating behaviors. I thought I was the only one that did bizarro things like that! (I'm not throwing donuts out the window, but you know what I mean.)

Like my friend, do you eat in shame? Instead of suffering in the dark, come out into the light where I can see you. Hear my loud voice when I reveal this startling truth: *You are not alone.* Even if you aren't spitting pastries into a bag, I'm guessing that you have a few eating secrets of your own that you'd prefer not to share. We all have skeletons in the closet. There is nothing you haven't done that someone else reading this book hasn't done, too. *There is nothing wrong with you; you are not a bad person.* The first step in helping you heal your wounds, though, is to figure out *why* you might be using these behaviors.

See if you recognize some common emotional states that lead you to overindulge (especially when you're not even hungry):

Emotional Triggers

- Anger
- Anticipation
- Anxiety
- Boredom
- Depression
- Desire
- Excitement
- Exhaustion
- Grief
- Joy
- Loneliness
- Nervousness
- Sadness
- Stress

It might be surprising that positive feelings of joyfulness, anticipation, or excitement are common triggers for over-eating. Just like with anger or depression, extreme emotions make us feel off-kilter. We long for internal equilibrium—to get back to "normal." When we eat, dopamine is released in the brain and provides a calm feeling that gets us back to stability again. Like any drug addict, we crave this physical reaction from food.

Emotionally, we've been programmed to lean on food for support. Feeling sad? Eat a cookie. Depressed? Have some chips. Intellectually, we know eating these foods won't make us feel better in the long run, but we all feel psychologically tempted in the moment . . . *because it works (for just an instance!).*

For some reason, one story comes to mind when I think about this topic. Years ago, when I was at my heaviest, I remember traveling overnight for work. I was feeling very isolated in my hotel room, and to kill time, I slipped out to a bakery for a late-night snack. Almost in a shroud of secrecy, I slinked back to my hotel room with a family-sized slice of carrot cake. I missed my family terribly and felt worried about my new job. Perhaps I hoped the cake would wipe away my feelings of loneliness and stress?

The reason this story stands out in my memory, though, is that I remember *exactly* how I felt *before* taking the first bite. *I became sad, really sad, that soon, the cake would be gone.*

This was an "aha" moment. For the first time, I admitted to myself that once the dessert was gone—"*poof*"—the magic would be over. I understood how the cake would only soothe my emotions *while I was actually eating it.* I realized the comforting feeling provided from the cream-cheese frosting would be short-lived, *but interestingly, I ate it anyway.*

Swallowing the Pain

Experiencing a major life change is often the impetus for gaining significant amounts of weight. After reading thousands of letters from my readers, I noticed this common trend. They swallowed their pain, quite literally, until things got out of control. Many of their stories overlapped. Here are the most popular triggering events:

- Auto accident
- Chemotherapy
- Chronic illness
- Death of a loved one
- Divorce
- Financial trouble
- Infertility
- Job change
- Medical issues
- Medication changes
- Miscarriage
- Moving
- Pregnancy
- Relationship problems
- Smoking cessation
- Unemployment

Food is such an effective distraction. When big problems come our way, like with a job or relationship change, eating starches and sweets seems like the best course of treatment!

FACEBOOK SHOUT-OUTS

Emotional Eating Stories from the DLK Support Group

"I wasn't prepared for the empty space that was left when I started DLK. For so many years, eating and time with friends always went together. It surprised me to figure out that food means more than just nutrition. I've learned I need to plan more activities with friends or I start to feel lonely when I eat." —Kimberly

"Happy. Sad. Excited. Anxious. Angry. No matter what I'm feeling, I pair it with food!" —Brad

"I gained more than sixty pounds last year when I quit smoking. I get antsy and just start eating. It's not like I'm hungry or anything." —Cynthia

"My weight issues really got out of control when we were trying to get pregnant. I have Polycystic Ovarian Syndrome (PCOS) and struggle with infertility. I always turn to sweets when I feel depressed." —Deb

"I've been on and off medication for years to help me cope with depression. When I feel anxious, snacking helps calm me down." —Barbara

"When my job gets stressful, I end up eating carbs like Pac-Man." —Leslie

The problem, however, is when we go overboard, especially with high-carb desserts, to calm ourselves down. Have you noticed that no matter how much sugar we eat, our dark emotional holes are never filled? **Carbs beget more carbs; there is never enough to feel satisfied.** It's impossible to appease intense feelings by eating. To make matters worse, many of us rely solely on food to make us feel better. We have forgotten that there are actually many other ways to help ourselves cope with challenging situations. Nevertheless, we keep eating!

The key to weight-loss success is to identify the hot buttons. What emotions drive you to overeat? When you start to feel one of those triggers, stop and take a breath. Ask yourself, **"Besides food, what is it that I really want right now?"** How could this demand be met in a way that doesn't lead to overeating? Your motivation, if it helps you to reframe this, is to avoid self-destruction. You aren't trying to punish yourself by withholding chips. The transition to using something NEW to meet your needs is easier said than done, *I know,* but you have to start somewhere, right?

**What is food attempting to give you that
you might be able to get somewhere else?**

I realize these are pretty deep questions, and I suspect you don't have the answers to them on the tip of your tongue. I do want you to realize their importance, however. Really think about this issue and try to uncover your truth. Unlocking this puzzle is the secret to understanding obesity. *Once you figure out your answer (not someone else's!), you will finally be free to start healing.*

This process doesn't happen overnight. For me, there was a lot of frustrating trial and error. Grappling with how to fill my unmet emotional needs felt like the quest for the Holy Grail. I wanted to give up *many times.* While I searched for my own answers, I was tempted to take shortcuts. I certainly experimented with trying to speed ahead in the fast lane.

I hoped there was an easier way to lose weight. I didn't want to think about all this touchy-feely nonsense, which seems like a lot of work! There had to be a quick product to buy or some program I could just "sign up for," right? I searched high and low for magic snake oil.

Nope. No such luck.

I did learn, however, that supplemental "solutions" were often effective as a stopgap. At first, some of these weight-loss strategies worked as fast as Amazon Prime. They delivered gifts of easy, fast weight loss. *Or so it seemed.*

As the queen of taking the easy way out, I was desperate for cheap and disposable solutions. It was a sad day, though, when I realized these topical solutions were just Band-Aids that would fall off after a short time. They didn't address the underlying, long-term emotional issues that made me overweight. Worse, some only "worked" when strictly followed but then backfired with *weight gain* afterward. *That's so not fair.* I'm confident you will recognize strategies on this list; I know I've tried just about all of them myself!

Let's take a look at commonly used, often flimsy short-cuts:

Fast Lane to Weight Loss?

CONTESTS and CHALLENGES—Using "thirty-day challenges" or similar weight-loss initiatives to motivate us to change behaviors, which last only for a short length of time.

DISTRACTION—Keeping busy, changing one's environment to avoid food.

MIMICKING—Copying someone else's prescribed meal plan instead of learning to independently prepare foods and make educated choices; using prepackaged shakes/bars, purchased meals, or eating only one food for a prescribed amount of time (e.g., an egg fast).

NEGATIVE REDIRECTION—Rerouting food impulsivity toward other equally self-destructive behaviors, like gambling, smoking, using drugs, abusing alcohol, or exhibiting hypersexual behavior.

POSITIVE REDIRECTION—Replacing food impulsivity with obsessive, over-the-top behaviors directed toward a replacement activity (finding religion, practicing extreme exercise, adopting a new "cause").

SCHEDULING—Setting strict times for "allowed" eating, like with intermittent fasting, fasting, or OMAD (one meal a day).

SUBSTITUTE FOODS—Finding alternate comfort-food recipes or products (e.g., low-carb ice cream).

WISHFUL INTERVENTION—Looking for a "magical" solution from a pill, shot, ketone drink, supplement, or medical procedure.

Too often, we convince ourselves that simple food substitutes will do the trick. When I'm feeling nervous, for example, I want to munch on something to calm myself down. Eating is my first instinct, *which, I'll admit, often works.* Instead of wolfing down high-carb chips, I've learned to just change the snack to something like celery or to chewing sugar-free gum instead. My nervousness is instantly cured, right? Sometimes, yes. But when a piece of gum quickly morphs into the whole pack, one piece after the next (*yes, I'm aware that this is kind of embarrassing!*), I know I'd better wake up. When this kind of binge behavior rears its head, I know my emotional needs warrant further attention. A single piece of gum isn't going to cut it!

Our feelings are a complicated business. When we don't acknowledge them, they tend to keep popping up—sometimes in unexpected ways. It's like a game of Whac-a-Mole. Just when you think you've successfully hammered down a feeling, it pops back up in a different way. Remember that anxiety I mentioned earlier? My body gets angry when I don't acknowledge when it's feeling stressed. When I attempt to suppress my feelings with a piece (or pack) of gum, my anxiety often escalates. Eventually, if I continue to ignore my stress, it manifests from just a feeling into a physical form. It doesn't ever go away.

I'm Stressed Out!

Often, these physical "giveaways" alert me that my stress levels are out of control:

- Clouded thinking
- Diarrhea or stomach issues
- Headache
- Heart racing
- Illness
- Insomnia
- Obsessive thoughts
- Psoriasis
- Tiredness

Deal with It

My wise friend Tamara (and DIRTY, LAZY, Girl podcast* cohost!) is always willing to do the hard work when it comes to addressing her feelings. I really respect her attempts to "go deeper," to address what's really going on with her feelings. (She doesn't just reach for a DIRTY, LAZY, KETO snack like I usually do—*which is always my first instinct.*) We like to brainstorm other ways to deal with our feelings and then report back to each other about whether they were effective or not. I'm going to share our ideas with you here. There

---

* *DIRTY, LAZY, Girl* podcast by Stephanie Laska and Dr. Tamara Sniezek. Links to listen and subscribe are available at https://dirtylazyketo.com/podcast-2/

is no one-size-fits-all way to handle our problems, that's for sure. Depending on what you are dealing with and your personality type, I'm sure you'll benefit from one or more of these techniques. Ultimately, we need an arsenal of coping practices, even those that look "hokey"! Take a risk and try something new. You might be surprised at how valuable these strategies can be in supporting your weight-loss efforts.

Suggested Strategies to Clarify Emotions

ART THERAPY—Explore feelings through nonverbal creative outlets (such as drawing, painting, craft-making, or creating sculpture).

EXERCISE—Engage in activity and movement to help the body process and liberate pent-up emotions.

MEDITATION—Release feelings through patterned breathing, visualization, or prayer.

MUSIC THERAPY—Play an instrument to express emotions.

NATURE—Enhance vitality and a sense of well-being by spending time outdoors. Connecting with nature restores perspective and improves mood.

PET THERAPY—Trust an animal to provide comfort and companionship.

SILENCE—Enjoy calming, quiet hobbies that don't muffle your inner voice.

SLEEP—Prioritize and engage in a regular sleep schedule to improve physical capabilities.

SOMATIC METHOD—Feel and acknowledge where physical stress is manifested (like in your posture,

different muscle groups, or facial expressions),
allowing your stress to be "heard."

TALK THERAPY—Share your feelings out loud with a
trusted friend, professional, or in an appropriate
support group.

VOCALIZATION—Sound out your emotions through the
flow of songs, chants, or mantras.

WRITING—Channel thoughts through journaling, writing
poetry, or creating song lyrics.

Is She for Real?

These strategies have turned my life around. I'm betting there
are some concepts here that can help you, too! These strategies won't cure overeating—*I wish it were that easy*—but they
will give you alternatives for hitting the vending machine.
All this gobbledygook is from my own playbook. THESE are
the newfound strategies I'm trying to use in place of overeating. Some of them have been more effective than others, for
sure. I struggle implementing some of them (like meditation
or getting enough sleep), even though I know it would be
helpful. It's easier to focus on the familiar. I certainly have
my favorites!

Combining the strategy of exercise with time in nature has
proven to be the most effective stress-management tool in my
arsenal. There isn't a problem in the world that I haven't been
able to solve by going on a run. I experience mental clarity, or
a "runner's high," when I'm out hitting the pavement. No, I'm
not lying right now. This is a real phenomenon! Everything

in my life *just makes sense* after finishing a run. *If that's not motivation to lace up your shoes, then I don't know what is!* Interestingly, I don't get this feeling when I'm indoors running on a treadmill. There is something magical about running outside in the fresh air that improves my mood. I'm reminded that there is a whole big world out there. By spending time with nature, my problems are put into perspective and become almost inconsequential.

If I'm not outdoors running, then I'm walking and talking. My dog-walking buddy, Tamara, and I log regular "counseling" sessions by combining outdoor exercise with the baring of souls. I depend on friendships like hers to support me through ups and downs. It's not that my friends have all the answers; that's not the case at all. But I do rely on their support. I need consistent, safe outlets for self-expression. Whether it's through talking to my dog, Lulu, or silently writing out a blog article to share with my Facebook support group, **releasing my feelings keeps me from eating them.**

Don't be afraid to try a new strategy. Yes, it might feel uncomfortable at first, because you don't know what you're doing, or you might feel "bad at it." It's natural to want to stay only within your comfort zone. But I urge you to push through. The benefits of adding new tools to your arsenal outweigh the fear of taking risks. *You don't have to be perfect to be successful, remember!*

A year ago, I challenged myself to learn how to play a musical instrument. I was inspired after watching my son take guitar lessons. I was so intrigued that I started futzing around with a ukulele. After watching hours of YouTube videos, I learned how to jam with only a handful of chords.

Surprisingly, I've fallen head over heels in love with this instrument! I even joined a club in my community that holds monthly sing-alongs to motivate me to practice. My romance with the ukulele is *not* because I have any talent; *that's* for sure. Instead, I love the way it makes me feel. **Singing, while playing music, wakes up my soul: I feel joyful, young, and optimistic.** I never experienced that kind of happiness from eating a bowl of popcorn!

Know Your Limits

When our urge to overeat stems from more serious issues, we must ask for outside help. Don't be afraid to find one-on-one professional support or join group therapy to get you through dark times. This doesn't mean you are weak; it means you are human. There is nothing to be embarrassed about. I know I've said this before, but it's important you hear me. *You are not alone* in what you are going through. *This is not your fault.* It might feel like it, but let me assure you that there are plenty of others in your same situation. You don't have to deal with this alone. There is help for you. If you recognize yourself involved with anything on the following list, please realize that your problem is bigger than what you are capable of handling on your own.

- Alcoholism
- Domestic violence
- Drug addiction
- Eating disorders: anorexia, bulimia, binge-eating

- Extreme grief
- Feeling out of control
- Self-harm
- Severe depression
- Sexual abuse
- Spousal abuse
- Suicidal thoughts
- Thoughts of harming others

If you are experiencing any of these issues, you need to ask for help—*right now.*

There is a way out of this mess, I promise. You can do this, my brave friend: ask for help. Your life might even depend on it.

You can't keep stuffing your feelings down with food, hoping your problems will "go away." No matter how big or small, your emotions will keep bubbling up to the surface. We all experience feelings of guilt, shame, embarrassment, and fear related to our weight problems; you are not alone! There are other ways to soothe your pain.

Find Your Voice

Self-care and managing your feelings are at the heart of finding your path for weight-loss success. There is no quick fix. If there were an easier way to lose weight permanently, I think we would all line up and sign over our firstborn. (*Sorry, kids.*) Learning to process our emotions, the permanent solution to avoid weight problems, feels so darn *complicated*. Nobody wants to admit this is true! Yet, despite knowing this is our best tool to fight obesity, we continue to drown our every emotion with food. *Why is that?*

Some of us don't feel worthy of acknowledging our feelings to begin with. Women, in particular, often feel their needs or feelings don't matter. Whether stemming from cultural messages or familial upbringing, from the time we are little girls all the way to adulthood, women hear a chorus of voices telling them to "be quiet" and "do what you are told." That, my friends, is some serious baggage women need to overcome.

Finding your voice isn't the only obstacle; it's just the beginning. Once you do speak up, you'll undoubtedly find that confronting issues is NOT fun. It can be embarrassing, painful, and awkward to discover what's *really* behind your overeating. You heard me right. I'm asking you to potentially feel *discomfort* instead of *contentment* from eating a yummy snack! (*Man, this girl is off her rocker.*)

"When we numb the pain, we also numb the joy."
—Brené Brown

Your emotions, both happy and sad, coexist simultaneously. Binge-eating temporarily dulls the pain, but at an extremely high cost. Anesthetizing despair by mainlining food unintentionally makes you unconscious of experiencing any emotion. It's not selective. **Gorging yourself blacks out everything: the good, the bad, and the ugly—*all at once.***

Once you stop numbing your "dark side," you'll be able to experience a full range of emotions. Ironically, suddenly "turning on the lights" in a previously darkened room can be the most liberating experience of your life.

By finally being able to see your fear and pain, you will simultaneously shed light on once-forgotten dreams, hopes, and desires.

It's time to release the glorious, joy-filled emotions accidentally swept under the rug. Behold! Feelings of passion, adventure, and wonder await you!

This experience will set you free from the shackles of obesity. Don't live in the darkness even one second more. *What you discover will be the greatest surprise of your life.* Aren't you curious to find out what life has in store for you?

7

BUCKET OF CRABS

Dysfunction Support System—Compliments and Criticisms

As I've mentioned before, when I first started a DIRTY, LAZY, KETO way of life, I didn't tell a soul. This might seem counterintuitive to what's been recommended to you, but for me, this strategy worked. *Go ahead; keep it on the low-low!* It's really nobody's business what you're up to. In my opinion, you need time to figure this whole thing out before going public. It's a brave thing you are doing—trying to change your life—and sometimes that decision needs to be made *in private*. Plus, you'll quickly discover that folks can get maniacal, even "judgy" once they discover you're on (*yet another*) DIET.

People react in unexpected ways when they find out you are trying to lose weight. Friends immediately anoint you as their personal food priest or priestess and begin confessing. This happens to me *all the time*. (Truth be told, I don't need to hear what you ate for breakfast!) When you start looking sexy, spouses often get jealous. Coworkers might act indifferent and not say anything at all. Relatives pretend to be supportive but then immediately offer you a slice of cake. *Um, no, thanks.* In the movies, everyone is supportive of the main character desperately trying to improve his or her life. But in reality, people can become vindictive. Excuse my French, but sometimes *"Bitches be hatin'."* Misery loves company, and an ecosystem demands equilibrium. For these two reasons, when you begin to lose weight, people will generally FREAK OUT.

So, what are you to do—wear your skinny pants in secret? At some point, people around you pick up on the fact that you aren't eating their homemade lasagna or swilling margaritas at happy hour. I want to prepare you for what lies ahead, lest you fold under pressure and get pulled back to the carbolicious dark side. Despite the multiple layers of people whom you interact with (lovers, kids, parents, extended family, coworkers, neighbors, strangers), **there will be predictable reactions to your weight loss.** By becoming familiar with their likely feedback, you won't be caught off guard.

Have you ever seen a *bucket of crabs* pulled from the ocean? The crabs will actually climb over each other, forsaking all existing relationships, with the goal of climbing out of the bucket—it's survival of the fittest! What makes this analogy so interesting, however, is that the remaining crabs inside the bucket work together, *antagonistically,* to prevent the hero crab from escaping.

"Not so fast!" they seem to shout while grabbing your leg. "You're not crawling out anytime soon!"

The same behavior can be expected from folks in your day-to-day life. With more than two-thirds of adults weighing in as overweight or obese in America, I'm betting the majority of people in your immediate circle also struggle with their weight. You might naïvely expect that because your cohorts are also plus-sized, they will sympathize with your issues and become your biggest cheerleaders. *Sadly, this couldn't be further from the truth.* In actuality, it's been my

"Every week at church people comment on my weight loss. I've heard everything from 'You look too skinny—eat this,' to 'Keto makes you get high cholesterol.' It's like they think it's their duty to inform me of the right way to eat. I almost don't want to go to church anymore." —Margaret

"Nobody cared when I was fifty pounds overweight and eating Pop-Tarts for breakfast, but now that I'm eating keto, everyone has an opinion!" —Diego

experience that most people fall into the "bucket of crabs" category. Perhaps covertly, without consciously knowing the power of their words, their needling criticisms and backhanded compliments seek to sabotage your hard work. Don't let them pull you back into the bucket of crabs!

Why does this happen? When you start to make healthy changes, people can feel threatened. Without your saying anything out loud, your actions criticize the behavior of those around you. When a crablike "friend" proclaims, "You've been so good, have a piece of cake with us," they are really saying, "I want to eat cake myself, BUT if *you* don't eat a piece, too, *I'll* feel guilty."

Crablike behavior isn't always easy to spot; it's often masked with kindness.

"You look fantastic; you don't need to lose another pound!" might be enough cause for you to slip back into old habits. Similarly, you might observe silent but destructive activity from those you share a kitchen with. When a spouse taunts you with sugar treats, either by stocking them in the fridge or by eating unhealthy foods in front of you, he or she is slowly but surely attempting to pull you back into an extra-large coffin of obesity.

As you lose weight, you may lose some friends, too. This really surprised me, and I fought it for a long time. It's kind of sad, really, that some friendships won't survive the "new you." Some people become overly jealous, but others just won't tolerate change. I was surprised how routine and familiarity were more important than my friendship. A close friend said goodbye to our decade-long relationship because I no longer shared a love of refillable popcorn tubs at the movies. Don't get me wrong, I still sneak an entire backpack of treats into the movies, but my contraband now consists of low-carb options. I smuggle packets of nuts, olives, celery sticks, and seltzer water instead of dollar-store candy, Mountain Dew, and microwaved popcorn. Even though I didn't make a big deal over my new eating choices at the cinema, the sound of my crunching on celery *literally and figuratively* led my friend to choose a different, long-standing movie date, "for-evah." Sad.

The mentality of the "bucket of crabs" extends beyond your home. At my work, I observe most women regularly lunching on light meals, like simple salads. This makes sense, as I work in the health-care industry, and most of my colleagues are petite health nuts. There was one gal, however, who, like me, stood out from the crowd with her lunch order. She loved eating her cheeseburgers, fries, and Coke! My hungry friend religiously sat next to me at mealtime, making snide comments about the dainty, meager choices made by our coworkers. Since I was ordering manly, extra-large meals for myself, I think it made her feel better to enjoy her full-sized platter while sitting next to me at the table. We were in it together, dining without care, concern, or an ounce of guilt. As I started losing weight and changing my eating choices, however, there was an abrupt change in our relationship. When my friend overheard me ordering something "healthy" the next time we were eating out, she made a pouty face and abruptly revised her order to a carb-lite meal more similar to mine. This didn't last long, however. Soon she avoided sitting next to me at lunchtime altogether. Her avoidance felt confusing to me.

Facing the bucket of crabs can make you feel alone and awkward. When norms or "routines" change, it feels un-comfortable to everyone involved. As a result, you might be tempted to cave "just this once" to ease the tension. *Don't do it!* Missteps like this contribute to failure. Rather than caving to the pressure, addressing awkward moments like these head-on will be a milestone in your weight-loss jour-ney. Merely recognizing *when* they are happening is a cause for celebration. *Baby steps will lead you toward success, even when they occur at a snail's pace.*

Weight-Loss Casting Call

Not everyone will become a "hater." There *are* some kind souls out there. When you find legit cheerleaders of your weight loss, invite them to join you inside your *circle of trust*. Building a sturdy, robust support system, whether it consists of a trusted therapist, online support group, or a well-intentioned friend, is absolutely imperative for sustainable weight loss. *You cannot, I repeat, cannot skip this step.* You need your "peeps" to support you as you embark on the most daring chapter of your life.

When I started this plan, I chose not to share it with my mom. That was a wise decision. I didn't bring it up, and neither did she (even as it became really obvious!). My weight is a loaded topic from my childhood, and I decided I didn't want to revisit that drama. Here I am 140 pounds *and seven years later* and the elephant in the room STILL has not been acknowledged. This is my choice. Finally, as a grown-ass adult, I've realized this is *my life*; I get to *choose* who enters my circle of trust. Maybe your family is screwed up, too; you might also blame your parents for your weight problems. Unfortunately, you can fault them all you want, but the blame game won't help you lose weight now. This is your deal and you're stuck with it. You have to take it from here.

That's not to say I don't sympathize. I've been on diets since second grade. My parents tried to bribe me to lose weight at a young age by dangling smaller-sized Jordache jeans as the reward. I was only eight years old, people—*no wonder I am having problems as an adult!* Was I doing the grocery shopping in elementary school, planning meals, or stocking the kitchen? No way! I didn't even pack my own lunch back then. My weight was a constant topic of conversation between my mother and grandmother. My weight and food choices were *constantly* being critiqued.

You may not be able to choose your family, but you can choose whom to discuss this topic with. Choosing whom you admit into your circle of trust is entirely within your control.

#BreakTheRules

When you venture outside of your circle of trust, I recommend you wear body armor for protection. Prepare for battle, my friend! Everyone feels the need to become your personal kitchen sheriff when you change your eating habits. The (self-appointed) food police will snarl at your food choices and offer a running commentary on what you *should* or *should not* eat. Their motivation might have the best (*or worst!*) intentions, but either way, food police are super annoying. I give you permission to nod your head, smile, and pretend to listen, all the while fantasizing about giving the food police officer a well-deserved *bitch slap*. Eating a DIRTY, LAZY, KETO lifestyle is controversial to some, and you should be prepared to either argue until you're blue in the face with charts and medical journals, or simply smile and let your coworkers lecture you on why a low-fat diet is superior (*which it is not!*).

Not everyone will have the cojones to question face-to-face your new way of eating. Some prefer only to comment on your weight loss politely *behind your back*. The *avoiders* will run from you and avoid eye contact at all costs. They are likely overweight themselves, and seeing you make positive strides toward better health makes them think about their own shortcomings. If your avoiders are close friends or family members, their actions (or lack thereof) can be extremely painful

FACEBOOK SHOUT-OUTS

Huh? Unexpected Reactions

Stories from the DLK Support Group

"I've lost ten pounds, but no one says anything. I feel so discouraged. I finally asked my husband why he hasn't said anything, and he said I always look nice." —Deb

"My best friend pretends not to notice I've lost almost thirty pounds. She hasn't said a thing! When I try to talk about DLK, she changes the subject. I don't even want to hang out with her anymore." —Tracy

"People keep saying 'nice outfit' or 'nice hair' to me. I don't think they realize I've lost weight. It's like they're confused when they look at me. Kind of funny, really!" —Jada

"Everyone in my family used to give me a hard time when I was overweight. They constantly made comments about my size. Now that I'm on the keto train and finally losing weight, they tell me I look too skinny and should stop. My dad even said I look sick. I'm so confused—I still have fifteen more pounds to lose before I'm even out of the overweight category!" —Melissa

"I stopped joining my coworkers in the break room because all they want to talk about is the way I look and how much weight I've lost. It's embarrassing. I'm a private person." —Eric

"My friends keep saying I deserve a night off from keto when we go to happy hour." —Paul

"If your husband is anything like mine, he tells you he supports you being healthier but complains when you don't buy cookies at the store." —Lori

and confusing. Compassion and patience are prescribed in heavy doses here. Give the avoiders time and space to come around.

The *nice-to-meet-you crowd* is indignant. They pretend not to notice your changing shape for whatever reason. Maybe they just don't care or are too self-absorbed to pay you a compliment. Sometimes, people don't say anything because they feel it isn't polite to talk about your weight issues. Either way, they talk to you (every time) as if nothing has changed. I have to admit, their behavior is so weird! It's important to be aware of how you are feeling during encounters when people appear to ignore your weight loss. Were you expecting a reaction and didn't receive one? Are you now feeling down about yourself and worrying your weight loss isn't "enough"? Rather than dismiss any feelings about being ignored, allow your internal conversation to play out. Be confident with your accomplishments and remember *some people suck*. It's important to connect with your feelings during the weight-loss journey. This process isn't easy! In fact, losing weight takes you on an emotional roller coaster full of dizzying highs and unexpected lows. If you find yourself feeling full of doubt, let me reassure you: *You are enough!* You do look fabulous. You are on the road to success, whether the nice-to-meet-you crowd notices or not.

The *fan club*, of course, is my favorite. Who doesn't love compliments and support? This losing-weight business is hard work. Sometimes, however, it can be downright embarrassing or even distracting to receive a compliment. One morning I was at yoga class with a friend who was struggling to lose weight and was having some success. In the middle of our crow pose, the instructor interrupted the group zen by pointing at my friend and loudly exclaiming, "Wow! You've lost so much weight that you can finally do this pose!" My yoga partner was humiliated and mortified. She wanted to crawl under her yoga mat to disappear. Because of this experience, she never returned to that class again.

Be aware that compliments don't always make you feel flattered. Some might lead you to feel ill at ease, causing you to revert to old eating habits to self-soothe. When you are heavy, you are often invisible to the world. Losing weight suddenly turns a spotlight on you. The attention can be unnerving. My yoga friend told me that compliments cause her to experience feelings of panic: she is afraid of others seeing her weight loss because then she feels added "public pressure" *not* to gain it all back.

On the flip side, the fan club might appear in disguise, in the form of *mean girls and guys.* A backhanded compliment might seem polite on the surface but stings upon further reflection. "I'm so glad you finally decided to lose weight—you look so great now!" makes you feel pathetic about previous stalled attempts and makes you worry you were unattractive to the world all along.

Take stock of how you're feeling when mean girls and guys appear. Fan club members can waiver between being helpful or hurtful. Criticism masked as compliments can send you running toward food for solace. Recognize when this happens and call out the BS that it really is. You do not want to derail your success. Practice self-assurance. Be loud and proud about your triumphs and speak up for yourself. *Fight back*. Cut these people loose.

Ugh . . . Change is hard. You'd think changing eating habits would be the hardest part of the weight-loss riddle, but in my experience, that part was the easiest. That portion (get it?) was cut-and-dried. Learning to stop numbing my feelings with food and to navigate relationships was *much* more complicated.

Some of my challenges may seem silly, I know. But let me ask you a question before you pass further judgment. Have you ever lost a significant amount of weight, but then gained it right back? Why do you think that happened? Maybe it wasn't your fault.

The strength of our support network (or lack thereof) is your greatest predictor of maintaining weight loss.

Friends and family unknowingly can derail your progress by saying things like, "You can have just one," or they insist, "You look just fine!" Stop sabotage with firm resistance.

With kindness and compassion, *tell your loved ones exactly what you need for support,* as it may be just blind ignorance or old habits guiding their behavior. Build a war chest of *real* supporters. Strong backing is vital for your ability to succeed!*

How to Show Support—Homework for Your Family

- Ask, "What can I do to help?"
- Validate her feelings with sincere empathy.
- Listen.
- Give sincere compliments.
- Tell him you are proud.
- Leave written notes of encouragement.
- Acknowledge these changes are hard.
- Have patience.
- Use encouraging, positive words about her lifestyle change.
- Eat and/or cook new recipes with him.
- Notice when she updates her appearance (like a new hairstyle or makeup).
- Be open-minded about new foods in the house or on the table.
- Stock the fridge with DIRTY, LAZY, KETO foods *without being asked.*
- Support special requests at restaurants: "No, he did not order fries; please bring the side salad instead."

---

* I host a free, large support group on Facebook: https://facebook.com/groups/dirtylazyketo. And for those wanting a smaller, more intimate group: https://www.facebook.com/groups /DIRTYLAZYKETO.Premium.

- Be patient at restaurants when she is learning how and what to order.
- Focus on positive progress (i.e., do not focus on her mistakes or setbacks).
- DO NOT eat high-carb foods (chips, ice cream, etc.) in front of him.
- Suggest activities to do together that don't trigger food cravings (like going for a walk).
- Notice small changes as they happen (i.e., do not wait until goal weight is achieved).
- DO NOT order dessert (or foods that tempt her).
- Support money to be spent on self-care, new clothes, and healthy foods.
- Relocate tempting high-carb foods away from his sight.
- Do not judge when she make a mistake.
- Reserve criticism.
- Compliment his weight-loss efforts to others (especially when he isn't around).
- Spend extra time at the grocery store to read labels and buy the "right" foods.
- Remind her you will always be there, no matter what she weighs.
- Celebrate achievements with him in ways that don't include food.
- Learn about her new way of eating: ask questions.

Your changes in eating habits will cause others to look at their own self-indulgent behaviors. Expect some folks to fight back either with smiles on their faces, silently, or with inappropriate comments. Your weight loss can be intimidating. Rest assured, however, that you are doing something incredible by making positive changes to your life. Your friends may not be in the same place as you. When you are brave enough to make a change, you lead by example, and not everyone is ready for that.

True friends will evolve with you. For some, this might take time. If you have a friend who is struggling with the "new you" but still kind and supportive about your new ways, help the relationship change. Find alternative ways to spend time together. Instead of your weekly date to watch a movie and eat buckets of popcorn, suggest a walk or take a class together. Give that friendship some space. Be patient. Let your changes sink in.

FACEBOOK SHOUT-OUT

Find Your Peeps!

Story from the DLK Support Group

"There are a few of us on DLK at work, so we started a lunch club! We made a schedule and take turns bringing in food like a potluck." —Summer

"I'm the only one in my family that struggles with weight issues. The Facebook support group is really the only place I feel comfortable getting help. I've made some great friends there, too." —Kai

On the flip side of this coin, you will make new friends. The "new you" will likely develop new interests. You might surprise yourself by making new friends. Remember my co-workers, ordering light, healthy meals at restaurants? I used to make fun of them, but now, I'm one of them. We have more in common than I realized.

True friends will support what you are doing and praise your accomplishments. When you encounter challenges, true friends will lift you up with encouragement. Utilize this support network by speaking up and talking through your problems.

Putting Theory into Practice

Logistically, day-to-day management of DIRTY, LAZY, KETO can sometimes get complicated. You might feel backed into a corner the first time you face a high-carb, high-pressure social situation. Other than asking your priest for a low-carb communion wafer, how will you survive?

Putting your sugar-free lifestyle into action might take some practice. Let's come up with strategies to help you get started. Yes, the first time you navigate the choppy waters, you might feel rudderless. Over time, though, the seas become easier to navigate. With practice, planning, and visualization, I'm confident you will soon be able to thrive in the most carbolicious of environments.

The Matador and the Bull?

Let's start with social situations, as these can be the trickiest. In my experience, whenever food feels "out of our control," one of two things is likely to happen. First, we grab the bull by the horns and take personal responsibility for the choices we make. I call this the Matador Approach. Whether you eat high-carb foods isn't the issue here. Matadors call the shots and make intentional choices. They stand strong and don't back down when faced with "danger."

Alternatively, take the easy way out and become the bull. With reckless, unplanned behavior, bulls break all the rules and convince themselves the damage was unavoidable, believing:

- "I couldn't help it."
- "It wasn't my fault."
- "There was nothing I could do."
- "I couldn't say no. That would be rude."
- "I was hungry and there wasn't any other choice."
- "I couldn't ask for special treatment from my hostess."
- "I didn't pick the restaurant."

You are certainly welcome to tell yourself these *bullshit* excuses (and many more, I'm sure). They sound soooooooo convincing when we say them to ourselves in the ring! But take a closer look at your "limited" options. There is always, I repeat, always, another way. It's one thing to *consciously* eat something carbolicious, but quite another to blame the decision on someone else or artificial circumstances. *You* are the one putting food into your mouth—no one else.

If you want a cookie, eat a damn cookie, but don't blame the Girl Scout who sold it to you.

I'd like to challenge your beliefs right now by asking an important question: **What would happen if you proactively and consistently made decisions that actually made you proud of yourself?** What if you were committed to your new lifestyle *no matter what*? Your answer is powerful. Listen to what you are saying! I can't do this for you, my friend. I can only show you the way. **You have all the power needed to achieve your goal.** DIRTY, LAZY, KETO works if you consistently follow the plan.

You're Invited! How to RSVP with DLK

Let's dive deeper and see how this all might apply to a specific example, like during the holidays. Every dieter on the planet lives in fear of the cold-weather holiday season. Halloween is just a warm-up event to test your commitment to weight loss. Next comes the main events—Thanksgiving, Christmas, New Year's Eve! Many Americans couldn't care less about the meaning behind these holidays; they only focus on the foods eaten to celebrate them. The deck is stacked against us from October through January. The holiday season is a worthy opponent of the DLK challenge!

Pretend you are invited to an informal holiday get-together. (Whether this takes place at work or home, it's all the same.) How do you respond?

RESPONSE A—Stay at home, feeling deprived, bitter, and angry that you can't "participate." While you might laugh at response A, I can see how it's sometimes an appropriate choice. When my friends got together after work at the bar for drinks and appetizers, at first, I needed to say no. I wasn't ready yet. I needed time and practice before I could make good decisions with a buzz on!

RESPONSE B—Show up. Eat everything that is served. Make many excuses to yourself about how you didn't have a choice. Feel guilty afterward. Continue circle of overeating/shame/weight gain. Eventually give up like you did on previous "diets." *I'm pretty sure 100 percent of us have fallen victim to this response at one time or another.*

RESPONSE C—Attend party but incessantly talk about your new DIRTY, LAZY, KETO lifestyle. Loudly criticize all the food that is being served and repeatedly complain there is "nothing for you to eat." Proceed to "educate" everyone about their terrible eating habits and demand special high-fat, low-carb food be served to you.

RESPONSE D—Show up and bring a dish to share, like any normal guest would do. Do you need to say anything about your dish? Nope. One of the beautiful parts about DIRTY, LAZY, KETO is that the foods look normal and taste absolutely decadent. No one will notice anything suspicious! Be sure you are first in line for the buffet as your dish might be gone by the time you get to it. In addition to enjoying the dish you brought to the party, enjoy low-carb, higher fat options commonly found at social gatherings: salad with dressing, fresh vegetables with dip, cheese, olives, meat—all washed down with water, diet soda, dry wine, Champagne, or a sugar-free cocktail.

Mingle, but keep current weight-loss plans to yourself. Calling attention to your new way of life might feel embarrassing. Unless you want to debate the merits of cholesterol levels on keto, I don't recommend making any grand announcements. *Not yet, anyway.*

HOW DID YOU RSVP?—How did you fare in this party scenario? Do you feel ready to venture out into the big, bad, carbolicious world yet? Some of these responses are comical, sure, but you can see how easy it can be to fall into a trap. If social situations have been your downfall in the past, take a pause and spend more time on this section. Practice and preparation are critical. Next, we will strategize practical tips for handling the party itself.

Party 101: Survival Tips

Strategy 1

Get involved in the party planning. Help the hostess plan venue options for the holiday dinner or party. Having the event at your own home or "cohosting" an event at another location will allow you more influence over the menu. If you are headed to a restaurant, take initiative by checking the restaurant's website for nutritional information (or call ahead to investigate what's on the menu). Whether a potluck or formal dinner, spend time beforehand planning out the exact steps you will take to be successful. Ask the waiter for a substitution, if need be. Make conscious choices about *where* you will eat, *what* you will bring, and *how* to enjoy your meal. Holidays don't have to become cheat days because they are "out of your control." Take responsibility for your health and enjoy the holiday, *but on your terms.*

Strategy 2

Make new dishes but keep the old. Holiday recipes are sacred. No one wants you messing with grandma's sweet potato pie recipe! Acknowledge the emotional element involved in family recipes. Sometimes people insist on a particular recipe because it reminds them of a family member who has since passed on. Is there an alternative way to honor your heritage? At my house we like to use vintage dishes and linens from long-gone relatives on "special occasions." These treasures help prompt fond memories and funny stories to keep the memory of those relatives alive. That being said, it's okay for you to contribute NEW dishes for the feast. There is nothing wrong with having multiple choices of a similar dish, like buttered green beans on one platter and green bean casserole with French's Crispy Fried Onions on another. Share a dish (or two or three!) that is on your DIRTY, LAZY, KETO plan.

Strategy 3

Prepare how to handle a potential backlash, big or small. Why? Because people can be controlling and downright emotional about their food choices. By bringing a new dish, or suggesting a new venue, a defensive hostess or family member might argue, "What is wrong with what I made?" In these situations, remind yourself calmly that it's them, not you, guiding their heated reactions.

It's easy to get caught up in this kind of "food drama." Emotionally charged conversations about the holiday meals alone might trigger a return to your old eating behaviors. Well-meaning relatives, the constant pressure to be "merry," and of course being presented with favorite comfort foods, can stall your weight-loss progress or, worse, cause utter derailment.

Strategy 4

Visualize the celebration in front of you. How do you "see yourself" at the event? Are you enjoying time with family, coworkers, or friends? Is there a tradition you enjoy at the event that you can look forward to? *Reframe your holiday to focus on traditions or activities, rather than food.*

Reframing the Holidays

Social events don't have to be a minefield for a DIRTY, LAZY, KETO way of life. With a little time spent on planning, practicing, and visualizing your holiday, you will thrive, not just survive, when faced with challenging obstacles. Holidays give us time to reflect, but are also an opportunity to start new traditions. When the meal is over and your relatives are carbo-crashed on the couch, you will be eating a second slice of sugar-free cheesecake and showing off your new skinny jeans.

8

PLANNING TO FAIL

Plan, Plan, Then Make Some More Plans

One of the most surprising discoveries I've had along my weight-loss journey is the need for a game plan when the shit hits the fan: *planning for failure is just as important as planning for success*. Bad things happen, that's to be expected, and a fresh-vegetable platter isn't likely to save the day. Whether it's financial trouble, a health scare, or family drama, there will always be something that can cause you to lose focus.

Not too long ago, I was a stay-at-home mom overwhelmed with two kids in diapers. I couldn't even take a shower without dragging a playpen into the bathroom. It didn't take long for my husband and I to realize we needed backup. For us, that meant moving closer to our nearest family members, who at the time lived over two hours away. Like many young married couples, we were overconfident about our financial future. Unfortunately, that naïveté translated into purchasing a home beyond our means.

When my husband lost his job, we didn't panic right away. We still had savings, good credit, and hope to rely on. I kept my chin up and a smile on my face, not admitting to myself or anyone else that we were in trouble. I continued to attend mommy-and-me playdates and toddler swim lessons. My husband went on multiple job interviews. Surely the tides would turn.

As weeks (and grim months) passed without any income, my buoyancy began to deflate. While the kids took afternoon naps, I ate. When they went to sleep at night, I drank. I didn't acknowledge my feelings at the time. Like any good midwestern girl, I kept my feelings private. Despite being terrified about my family's future, I said nothing.

Like my worries, my weight skyrocketed.

The Domino's Pizza delivery man started coming to my house as often as the newspaper. The warm half-calzone box was the crescent moon signaling the day had ended.

Around that time in my life, I remember putting the scale away because it "took up too much room" next to our toddler's potty chair. My husband asked where the scale went, and I responded in all honesty that it was broken (scales *do* stop working at three hundred pounds). I was in serious denial about what was happening to my weight. Even now, I feel ashamed to admit that I couldn't turn around all the way in my stand-up shower; I couldn't properly clean myself. Like a bad dream, much of the details during this time in my life are blurry. Is this fortunate or not? Alongside the painful reflections about our home's eminent foreclosure are the memories of my son taking his first steps and saying his first word, both of which I can't recall. Both the pain and the joy are literally blacked out in my mind.

Destructive Coping Mechanisms

Looking back, I think this was the saddest part of my marriage. This is not because we ended up losing our house—that's not it at all. It's because we hid in shame from what was happening. I may have been powerless over what was happening financially, true, but that shouldn't have silenced me. I needed to speak up! Bottling up my feelings, though it sounds so cliché, was the worst thing I could do for my health. Stress literally rotted my body from the inside out and drove me toward reckless eating. Instead of processing my fears, I swallowed my shame. I spent two long years drowning, with pizza as a life preserver.

My primordial response to pain was a desperation to feel better at any cost, to hell with the consequences.

Everyone has unhealthy ways of dealing with stress. I'm definitely not alone! Over the years, I've observed friends or coworkers distract themselves in equally destructive ways. They avoid facing their personal demons by turning to drugs, overspending, gambling, or cheating on their spouses. Everybody has their secrets! Unfortunately, my "go-to" coping strategy was difficult to hide: overeating shows up in added pounds.

I numbed my feelings with food. I'll be honest, eating made me feel good (still does), albeit only temporarily. I need to be hyperaware of when I feel the urge to revert to this perverse strategy. Better yet, I try to intervene before it starts. Whether it's with a trusted therapist, family member, friend, or through an online support group, I've learned how critical it is for me to unload my burdens by speaking up. Just saying my feelings out loud cleanses my spirit.

I've learned that I can survive just about anything if I have "my people" to help me get through it. By finding a friend to talk with, I feel better equipped to handle the stress in my life. I have to continually remind myself, though, to talk to a friend when I feel upset. It doesn't come naturally to me. Like a drug addict, my default coping mechanism will always be to turn to food first.

At the same time, I'm going to be realistic. I'm not going to set naïve expectations that I will always choose to talk through my problems first. That sounds exhausting and maybe idealistic! I'm pretty sure there will be times I'll cop out. Whether due to convenience or desperation, I expect there will be times I will still turn to food for comfort. *Are you surprised?* The difference, though, is that this choice is *deliberate.*

#BreakTheRules

Knowing how effective eating can be to manage my emotions, I sometimes make the conscious choice to—*gasp*—comfort myself with food. My intentional comfort-eating looks very different now compared to what it used to look like (different foods), but I still do it! Do I expect myself to be perfect? Nope! I'm probably a little broken, and I don't expect myself to ever be completely "fixed." Sometimes, I just want to self-soothe. Instead of a McDonald's vanilla milkshake, though, I'll make a sugar-free protein smoothie. The fast food straw, like an adult pacifier, calms me down. *Don't judge.*

By leaning into my proclivities, I've learned how working with myself, and not against, helps maintain my weight loss. These unlikely strategies, while so different from following conventional weight-loss advice, has helped prevent me from backsliding. That's good enough for me! *Maybe I don't have to "be perfect" after all, and certainly not all the time.*

These two techniques—sharing my feelings and willfully making substitute food choices when I eat for comfort—have helped me get through some very tough times. There will always be bumps in the road. The journey will never be completely stress-free. But now I feel more equipped to experience the ride.

> "Owning our story can be hard but not nearly as difficult as spending our lives running from it. . . . Only when we are brave enough to explore the darkness will we discover the infinite power of our light." —Brené Brown

Testing the Limits

My ability to handle adversity was thoroughly tested a few years ago when doctors found an ominous, softball-sized abdominal tumor weighing down my organs. I had been reporting backaches and abnormal menstruation to my doctor for over a year before a CT scan proved I wasn't just psychosomatic. Maybe I didn't complain loudly enough? I had numbed my body with food for so long that it's possible I didn't even know what physical discomfort felt like. Blood tests and radiologists confirmed I needed *immediate* major abdominal surgery, *like within days*.

My reaction might seem inappropriate, but when the oncologist told me I wouldn't be able to run (or lift weights, do yoga, or have sex) for many months after surgery, I didn't think about the possibility of cancer. In lieu of fearing for my life, my immediate response was worry over gaining weight. *Kind of pathetic, really!* Maybe I didn't want to think about eight body parts being removed (*eight!?!—didn't I need those parts?*), let alone any other potential ticking time bombs the surgeon could discover. I felt terrified. The situation was completely out of my control.

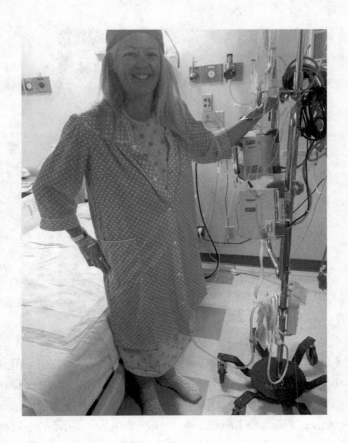

In order to push through my fears, I focused only on my part. If I ended up living through the ordeal, I was determined to come out the other side stronger. Maintaining habits of purposeful eating, consistent exercise, and projecting a positive attitude were my planned tools for survival. Yes, I allowed myself some pity-party time (*and a super cute new hospital gown*), but instead of eating donuts, I dyed my platinum hair the colors of the rainbow. I was going into battle on my own terms.

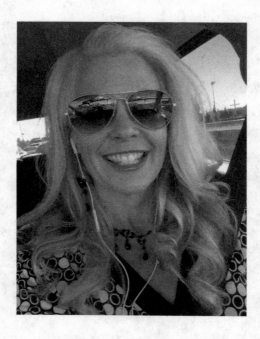

I didn't call Domino's for support, but I sure did call my friends. When I didn't feel comfortable saying my fears out loud, I jotted them down. I even wrote out my will. *Boy, that felt scary.* This might sound chickenshit, but I didn't exactly show anyone my will; I sent it in an email! I knew if I had to share it with anyone "ahead of its time" I wouldn't be completely honest when writing it.

Though it was probably not legally binding—*whatever!*—I emailed my last will and testament to my husband just before going into surgery. The subject line read, "open only if necessary." Whether he followed my directions about reading it, I'll never know, but including this caveat allowed me the freedom to honestly share my feelings *about everything and anything*. While normally I'm quite reserved with my emotions, there, in my e-will, I profusely thanked my husband for being the absolute love of my life. I got everything off my chest, even spelling out blessings if he were to remarry. Though morbid, I thought long and hard about the kind of funeral I would want: a luau celebration on Shipwreck Beach in Kauai after my ashes are illegally strewn into the Pacific Ocean. I imagined my family gathering around to say goodbyes with my favorite ukulele songs strumming in the background.

What if I survived the surgery and my illness? Would my continued existence be as romantic as my fantasized demise? Perhaps I needed a more practical plan beyond a *Fantasy Island* episode. In the past, bowls of Mother's Circus Animal Cookies and Blockbuster videos coaxed me back to good health. But this time, *this time,* I knew my approach would have to be different. I would tackle post-op care just as I would train for a marathon. I decided to make a recovery schedule. That's not super obnoxious or unattainable, *uh, right*?

The doctor thought my response was over-the-top, warning me that I had nothing to prove by planning such a speedy recovery. Sure, he was right, but I knew myself better than that. If I didn't have an aggressive plan for how to bounce back, I knew I might quickly revert to old habits. Being assertive about my health felt new to me. I didn't exactly have a strong track record for handling stress well. I needed to make a plan.

First, I committed myself to being accountable with daily exercise. While I knew I wouldn't be at water aerobics anytime soon, I anticipated being able to walk to the mailbox. I documented exactly how far I walked each day and proudly wrote down that number on a blank calendar page posted to the front of my refrigerator.

It might seem embarrassing for a marathon runner to write down "three laps around the nurse's station" for her first exercise entry, but writing down my achievements, no matter how small, motivated me to forge ahead.

Within weeks, under my doctor's supervision, I built up to an hour of walking every day. I was tired, sure; I would practically fall asleep as soon as I got home. Still, the walking helped my body *and mind* heal. My commitment to daily exercise reminded me that *I was still alive.* The fresh air gave me perspective and optimism. I felt happy. Just like with my previous weight loss, seeing incremental improvement on my accountability chart motivated me to push myself farther than if my efforts went unnoticed.

I'm not going to lie to you, recovery wasn't always a bed of roses. I didn't jump out of bed every single day, consistently motivated to lace up my running shoes. Sometimes I felt sore, exhausted, or just plain mad at the whole situation. But I didn't give in to my feelings of self-pity. I acknowledged my frustration, but went on to exercise anyway. **One of the tricks I learned during my weight-loss journey was the importance of relying on habits more than just motivation.**

Motivation is fleeting. I can be fired up to do just about anything for a short period of time, but those feelings aren't likely to be consistent. Motivation waxes and wanes over time; you can't depend on it. What I've found to be more reliable is to commit to an established routine. Before I had surgery, I religiously "worked out" first thing in the morning, Monday to Friday. (Weekends, I'm in rest mode, baby!) After my surgery, I decided to do the same thing. No, I wouldn't be running for an hour or lifting weights for activity, but I was confident I could *do something*.

I continued to lay out my workout clothes every night before going to sleep, just like I did before the surgery. My morning routine stayed the same. I woke up at the same time each day and immediately got dressed for exercise *no matter how I was feeling*. After eating a small breakfast, I left the house to "exercise." Like I said before, after my surgery, I used the term "exercise" rather loosely! I probably didn't need to be wearing a cute headband and matching running shorts for my slow crawl around the block, but maintaining the exercise schedule, cute outfit and all, meant I would stay consistent with the routine.

My friends were more than happy to support me, *once I asked for their help*. I was surprised that my running partner, Lori, continued to show up for our Monday workout (even though we wouldn't be running). I could only walk—not run—the five miles like we were used to. But she didn't give up on me! Tamara brought her dog over to walk with me and keep me company. She taught me how to download podcasts and made me laugh until my sides split, ultimately becoming my consigliere for all things related to DIRTY, LAZY, KETO. When things got too personal to share with my besties, I turned to an online support group of patients with a similar prognosis. Instead of stuffing down my feelings with Cheetos, I spoke them out loud or wrote them down, neutralizing their toxic powers.

In sum, I got better. It took more time than I'd expected for my abdomen to heal and for my hormones to stabilize, but I patiently plodded forward. My weight shifted here and there. I had to learn to manage the "new me." I modified my goals but stayed accountable to myself. To manage my roller coaster of feelings, I exercised and talked with friends. Having a plan and sticking to routines helped me survive, and ultimately thrive, during one of the most difficult times of my life.

Starting Over After a Whoopsie, a Whopper, or an Utter Fail

Success and failure are more closely linked than you might think. Planning how to celebrate weight loss is just as critical as laying out strategies to bounce back when things get tough. There will certainly be bumps, potholes, and *maybe road closures* along your weight-loss journey, and I want you to be ready for detours. No one said this was going to be easy, *just worthwhile!*

> **Starting over**—Kind of like going to rehab, sometimes it takes "more than one time" to try to lose weight

before we are fully ready to commit to a new lifestyle. No one is perfect. I want you to know that I'll support you *without any judgment*, as many times as it takes for this information to get through.

Weight-loss stall—Our bodies are complicated. Just because you are doing "everything right" doesn't always translate to immediate weight loss. Having patience, faith, and determination will get you through moments of frustration.

Unexpected weight gain—Hormone changes, illness, and medication can cause an unplanned increase on the scale. Eating foods with unfamiliar ingredients can also breed unexpected consequences.

Regretful decisions—It's normal to rebel and test your limits. This is part of what makes us human! I am constantly trying to see what I can get away with. If the decisions you make lead to feelings of regret, though, it's important to forgive yourself first before trying to refocus.

Lowered inhibitions—Alcohol and weight loss can be like oil and water if you aren't careful. After a stiff drink you may find that your willpower to make DIRTY, LAZY, KETO choices has diminished. For that reason, be hypervigilant when introducing alcohol to your weight-loss mix.

Cheat meal gone wrong—Even though you read my thoughts on "cheat meals," I'm sure there are a few of you out there who don't yet believe me. A cheat meal often expands to a cheat day, which then becomes a cheat month, or longer. If this happens to you, admit the truth about what went wrong and start again right now (*not tomorrow!*).

Climb Back on the Wagon

No matter what obstacles you face, know that you have the necessary tools to help you dust yourself off and jump back into the game. Mistakes, obstacles, or setbacks won't ruin all the work you've done *unless you choose to let that happen by continuing to cheat*. Sometimes a stumble helps prevent a fall. Learn from your mistakes, but, more important, forgive yourself for making them. Have the courage to be imperfect, my friend. This process is *not* easy.

9

BE VULNERABLE

Fear of Failure, Fear of Success: Is It Better Just to Hide?

Avoidance, Denial, and False Beliefs

For most of my life, sidestepping high-risk situations has been my foolproof method for avoiding embarrassment and failure. I figured if I didn't try something, I would never mess up! No wonder I never wanted to "start" another diet. Flunking yet another plan would be too humiliating. My history of numerous failed weight-loss attempts made me feel ashamed. I've been a successful person in every aspect of my life, but with my weight? I gave myself a failing grade. My attempts to reduce the number on the scale had belly flopped over and over again. I would lose weight, start to feel good about myself, but then backslide when someone reacted in an expected way.

Early in my twenties, I remember having some success on the Fat and Fiber plan from Weight Watchers. After losing twenty-five pounds or so, I thought I was ready to rock the world! My confidence took over the steering wheel, and I found myself driving to a local gym for a new-member orientation. (Other than taking an aerobics class with my mom at a local church, I had never been inside of an athletic club in my entire life!) The tour was going well until the perky nipple-head (this is what I used to call those gym rats with their hair on top of their heads in buns) asked me a question.

"What's your motivation for coming into the gym today?" she probed, hoping to gain insight for closing a membership deal.

"Uh, I've lost weight, and now I want to tone up?" I guessed.

"Right! You're still *skinny-fat*," the nipple-head assessed with a plastered, bleached smile.

Her words, though likely coached from a manager on how to "sell" a membership, cut to my core. Her "skinny-fat" comment made me feel completely ashamed about my new figure. I felt raw and out of place.

What was I thinking trying to sign up for a gym?!

Sadly, I smiled and agreed with her. On the inside, however, I was convinced she was right. My reduced weight *was still not good enough*. I did not belong at the gym and I would never be part of "the beautiful people," no matter how hard I tried.

Gym girls, with all their spandex, glitter, and giggling, seemed to be members of an exclusive club I could never be a part of.

However twisted, that was my mentality at the time. Sure, I had lost weight, but my self-esteem had not changed. Mentally, I was stuck in the past. I was angry and resentful about having to do all this "upkeep," like joining a gym. I didn't quite "get it" yet. I was so focused on changing the number on the scale, I forgot what was *actually* important—feeling good in my skin again. It's not surprising that I ended up gaining that weight back!

Overcoming a lifetime of bitterness wouldn't be easy.

When I moved to California as a teenager, I quickly realized that I didn't fit in. I realize this was due to my own hang-ups, but, boy, I harshly judged everyone around me! I remember getting so angry about artificially highlighted hair, athletic bodies, and fake tans. As if their orange skin was contagious, I avoided all contact with other students and referred to "them" as "*the Mannequins*." I didn't want to join their ranks; I convinced myself I was better than that. Maybe it was due to my immaturity, but as an adolescent, I believed I had only two *false choices*: to be plastic (and skinny) or real (and overweight).

I felt out of place compared to the Mannequins. I shopped in the plus-sized department, wore oversized baggy shirts, and sported elastic-waist pants. Maybe it was because of the cold weather in Michigan, but growing up, I felt most comfortable wearing flannel shirts or bulky sweaters. All girls want to look like fashion models, right? Well, apparently not me. My closet consisted of androgynous, "grungy" clothes (style of the 1990s). I didn't own a belt. I convinced myself for years that my style was rebellious, but if I'm being honest, I'm pretty sure I was secretly resentful about not having a stomach that could rock a crop top. Nonetheless, I hid my growing figure inside a wardrobe more fitting of a lumberjack than a college girl. I felt unattractive and awkward. Looking back, I imagine I might have just been hiding in those giant clothes just because I felt insecure.

People are constantly evaluating the way we look, whether we want to admit it or not. I'm not saying it's right or wrong. *Don't get your feathers ruffled!* I just want to point out that it's true. This is the world we live in. Because of this skewed reality, many of us, including me, have tried to lose weight with the goal of pleasing other people. It's a slippery slope, trying to look good for the wrong reasons; it's almost impossible to gain even footing when a motive like this is *just so wrong.*

I've wasted many years trying to change my weight for the wrong reasons. At times, I felt angry and spiteful. From dating to employment, I've been left feeling dismissed, rejected, and even invisible. My *first* husband, in one of our last fights before he left me for his secretary (sooooo clichéd, I know!), told me our marriage was ending because I had gained so much weight since our wedding, and as a consequence, I had become unattractive to him.

"You aren't the person I married," he sheepishly admitted, "and this"—*wagging his finger pointing up and down my body*—"THIS isn't what I signed up for."

Whoa—that was harsh!

Reader, you might be screaming at the page right now, hollering, *"HOW DARE HE, GIRLFRIEND!"*

Like you, my initial reaction was pain and, of course, ANGER. I wallowed in these negative emotions for a really long time. I falsely convinced myself that I would never find love or be attractive unless I wore a certain size clothing. I became blinded by this myth. It affected every aspect of my life.

I struggled to find work. I clearly remember a job interview that went haywire. I sat in an upscale hotel lobby waiting for my interview to start. I sat up straight with my legs crossed, wearing a pressed designer suit, hoping to make a solid first impression. When the hiring manager walked into the lobby just a few feet away, he only briefly glanced my way before scouring the rest of the room, looking for other possible candidates. In that moment, I sabotaged myself. I became convinced that the interviewer was not impressed that I was the next appointment. We were all alone in the lobby. I imagined a news flash before him: the lady in the blue suit *weighing close to three hundred pounds* was here to interview for the job!

I continued to get in my own way. I went on something like seventeen job interviews before finally getting my career started! Granted, I may have chosen a career path that relied more on "looks" than other types of jobs, but even as the most qualified and personable contender, I kept finding myself getting turned down. Was this due to my weight, or did I lack the confidence needed to get the job?

I'm sure you can relate to at least one of these stories. We've been conditioned to think being thin is synonymous with happiness, success, and romance. But in truth, the number on the scale is powerless. We can be capable, beautiful, and worthy of love . . . no matter what we weigh! The number on the scale just ends up being a reflection of our eating and exercise habits.

Fear, Embarrassment, and Trauma

Weight loss is not foolproof. Threats might be hiding around every corner. If you aren't prepared, you could get scared right back into your old carbolicious ways. I remember being surprised about the look of one such villain, as he was quite handsome and wore an unlikely red vest. This young man was a helpful employee in the electronics department at Target.

On a busy Saturday, I meandered over to the big-screen television section, hoping to elbow my way to a loss-leader sale item. I was greeted by a smiling stocker asking if I had any questions. This isn't unusual, I agree, except for the fact that there were tons of people ahead of me waiting in electronics for his help. I had just arrived, and this employee walked up to me straightaway, bypassing the crowd.

Why is he talking to me? I wondered. *Hmm . . .*

Despite the dirty looks and sighs from other customers, the young man proceeded to prioritize me as a customer. I was oblivious to the preferential treatment, but my young daughter was not.

She giggled and whispered coyly, "He keeps smiling at you!"

This memory stands out in my mind because it was the first moment when I noticed someone was treating me differently because of my weight—but in a positive way. I still blush thinking about that young man—*half my age!*—fawning over me like I was Mrs. Robinson. Interestingly, I remember having the most bewildered reaction. I *questioned* the attention, thinking to myself, "But I'm not thin yet," like

I didn't *deserve* his interest. I had lost about seventy pounds at this point, but in my mind "that didn't make me pretty"— *yet*. Isn't that sad?

"Looking good" (or not) to that red-vested gent wasn't the heart of the issue. This was about how I saw myself. This experience opened my eyes!

I realized that by focusing so much on the "outside," I neglected to work on what really mattered—my self-esteem. My body was changing, but my mind *was stuck*. If I didn't take action, I would continue to feel badly about myself no matter what I weighed. Chasing an arbitrary number on the scale (or having people notice me) was NOT the solution.

I had an "aha" moment, if you will—right there at Target, of all places. Losing weight was *not* the Holy Grail. How I felt about myself, *not a number on the scale,* was what I really needed to work on. I had to make that change in my brain. I needed to learn how to love myself . . . right *now*!

How much I weighed, getting a job offer, having someone be attracted to me—those weren't the real issues. I needed to love and accept my body at any size, at any age, through all stages of sickness and health. Only by figuring out how to become "body positive" would I ever win this battle. Achieving a healthier weight would be a by-product of self-love, not self-hate!

It's About You, Not Them

Experiencing weight-loss success is not all sunshine and roses. Receiving unwanted comments or advice from strangers can trigger acts of self-sabotage. It's confusing, to say the least. No one prepares you for how to handle the attention, both the positive *and* negative. When people questioned me about my weight loss, at first I felt embarrassed and had trouble answering. No matter what I said, people seemed to have a strong opinion about it. It was so bizarre. People seemed desperate to learn how I had lost so much weight, but they would then attack me once I told them how. In the end, I learned to just keep my mouth shut. Avoiding uncomfortable conversations like that kept me sane. I didn't need to explain myself to anyone, *right*?

I spent decades of my life hiding underneath black, box-shaped jackets and layers of fat. As those layers peeled away, there were unexpected consequences. People started to "see" me, and it felt, well, *weird*. I wasn't sure how to handle other people's reactions to the way I looked. In the end I realized "they" didn't matter. *I* was the only one I needed to please!

If you begin to feel defenseless, acknowledge it. Talk about your feelings with a trusted friend rather than letting emotions build up inside of you like in a pressure cooker. There is no way to avoid vulnerability. You can't run from it! Things come out eventually, and in destructive ways that you might not anticipate. You've got to process your feelings in a productive way that's under your control. Otherwise, the situation might turn on you. It's pretty common for self-doubt to grow during moments of vulnerability. This takes place in the form of counterproductive self-talk. You might even recognize some of these fabrications. Sadly, I think we've all caught ourselves saying these hurtful things to ourselves at one time or another.

Turn Off That Voice:
Destructive Internal Dialogue

"I'll never be able to keep this weight off; I should just give up now."

"I still look fat."

"I'll never get to my goal weight."

"My husband said I look just fine."

"Now there is so much pressure to keep this weight off."

"Everyone is saying I look too skinny and I should stop."

"Everyone keeps staring at me."

"This is too much work."

"It's too hard being the only one in my family eating this way."

"I need a break."

"I should be able to eat these foods like other people."

"This isn't working for me."

Trauma

Attracting attention can feel scary, too. I was surprised at how weight loss triggered upsetting memories. I struggled with whether or not to share this with you. I want to believe the DIRTY, LAZY, KETO message should only be lighthearted and positive, but the truth is that weight issues are often painful. There might be something in your past that is still getting in your way, too. I think it would be irresponsible for me to try to avoid this topic, because significant trauma affects so many of us with weight issues. After a lot of self-analysis, I realized my past trauma might be partly to blame for why I chose to conceal my figure with extra pounds over the years. I *didn't want* anyone looking at my body. I hoped an intentional shroud of fat might protect me from unwanted contact.

When I was younger, I was sexually assaulted. For years, I felt ashamed of what happened. It's taken me a long time to realize the incident *wasn't my fault*. Intellectually, I know the assault had nothing to do with my size. Being thin didn't make me likely prey, just like being heavy won't protect me from being hurt again. But I still struggle with this. To this day, I feel weird when men look at me or make a pass. I feel on edge, not flattered, by male attention. Being self-aware of my uneasiness has helped stop backsliding during my weight-loss journey. Instead of reverting back to old habits of overeating and gaining weight for protection, I try to face feelings of panic head-on.

Painful memories keep hurting if we don't resolve them.

To this day, I can describe in every aching detail about being taunted at summer camp. I remember not showering *for an entire week* after a fellow camper ridiculed my pudgy body while we were changing clothes. I refused to let that happen again, changing in the bathroom instead of in front of other campers and refusing to participate in the group showers. I dipped my pigtails in the water fountain to fool camp leaders that I had cleaned myself and washed my hair.

Without a doubt, every single person reading my story can recall painful instances of when they were made to feel disgusting, undeserving, or unlovable. Unfortunately, these memories tend to resurface during weight loss—be forewarned. Hearing positive compliments about weight loss, no matter how many pounds into your journey, simultaneously might bring up shameful feelings, like a double-edged sword.

"Have you lost weight?" sounded exactly the same to me as, *"Why were you so fat?"* It's a lot to grapple with, having these conflicting emotions.

During a time when you're feeling the most vulnerable, you undoubtedly will turn toward your closest relationships for support. But whether it's a best friend, parent, or spouse, what happens if this person isn't able to support you in a way that you need? Your beloved might not be able to help you. He or she might feel threatened because of your weight loss, or could worry you are trying to "move on" to someone or something else. I know this seems almost unimaginable, but because your loved one fears losing you, he or she might subconsciously retaliate and try to sabotage your weight loss.

While I don't want you to become an empathetic doormat, I encourage you to show compassion. Have patience. Give your family and friends time to adjust. Don't put up with hurtful interference, but provide assurance that you aren't going anywhere. In the meantime, take care of your needs. Find a support group. Seek professional help if need be.

You Are Smokin' Hot RIGHT NOW

Feeling body-positive takes practice. There are no shortcuts for this one. No "other" person is going to make you feel this way. Women tend to look outward for approval, so I caution you to "check yourself" if you see this happening. You most certainly need to *look inward instead of outward* for self-approval. This isn't as easy as it sounds. It takes practice! There is no better way to stoke your self-esteem than by practicing self-care and positive self-talk.

There is a myth about stepping on the scale that I'd like to debunk right now: reaching your goal weight won't change how you feel about yourself. Don't wait for your pride to magically explode at the finale of reaching your weight-loss goal. This isn't television. There will be no balloons falling from the ceiling! You've got to change the internal narrative you hear right now—not at the end. Ironically, losing weight will just be an added benefit to feeling great about yourself!

One of my favorite pictures ever taken of me was a selfie of my husband and me before a big race. I hadn't brushed my teeth yet and I wasn't wearing makeup, but I still felt absolutely beautiful. The rising sun was peeking up behind us over the Pacific Ocean, and we nervously waited at the starting line for the Monterey Bay Half Marathon. In the photo,

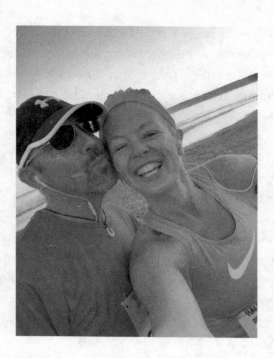

my bright smile and laugh is obvious. I felt strong, confident, and absolutely unstoppable. This moment marked months upon months of reprogramming the voice inside my head. I felt beautiful because I *finally received the positive message* that I had been practicing telling myself day in and day out for months. Not only did I hear the mantra, but in this moment, I *decisively allowed myself to believe it.*

Take Risks and Build Confidence

Entering the gates of Onederland* doesn't come with an automatic license to feel good about yourself again. You've got

---

* You enter Onederland when your weight starts with the number "one."

to work hard at building your self-esteem *every single day.* By taking chances and learning to feel vulnerable in a variety of situations, not just with weight loss, your self-confidence will slowly build.

Wearing a tank top, taking the lead at work, or simply admitting you need help—all have something in common. In each of these situations, you risk showing the world that you aren't perfect. Even in these ordinary examples, putting yourself "out there" to be judged feels a little risky (or maybe risqué, depending on what that tank top looks like!). It's scary to live our best life. Sitting on the couch is undoubtedly safer. The rewards from adventure are only possible, though, if you take chances to begin with. Opening yourself up to being vulnerable won't make you weak. Ironically, trying new things, especially if you stumble or fall, is actually what makes you stronger.

Taking risks and learning to become resilient means you are living to your full potential.

I'm so committed to this belief that I now use vulnerability as a litmus test for personal growth. If an activity makes me feel uncomfortable, I give it *tenfold* the consideration. I recently had the opportunity to choose between three activities: having a massage, playing a round of golf, or ocean kayaking IN THE PITCH DARK. Can you guess which one I picked? Sure, being naked in front of a stranger sounded pretty scary, but what about climbing in and out of a flimsy plastic boat *at night*?

Taking chances that push me *out of my comfort zone* have given me more joy, self-confidence, and happiness than anything I'd ever experienced before. Wearing a bikini, learning to play the ukulele, and even dyeing my hair pink **make me feel alive.** Running a marathon, riding a bike, writing a book . . . The list goes on. Sure, I might be criticized or laughed at. There might even be a loud chorus of "*Who does she think she is?*" in my wake. This is all true! What I say over my shoulder to these crabs trying to pull me back down is this: **I am choosing the bigger life.** Don't be scared. There is room for all of us.

Giving into self-doubt stonewalls me from experiencing the beauty life has to offer. Instead of constantly worrying about failing, I challenge you to flip that message on its head and I propose instead, "What if I *don't* fail at all? What will happen if I actually succeed?" *Maybe success, and not failure, is what I actually fear?*

"Our deepest fear is not that we are inadequate. Our deepest fear is that we are powerful beyond measure. It is our light, not our darkness, that most frightens us. We ask ourselves, who am I to be brilliant, gorgeous, talented, fabulous?"
—Marianne Williamson*

---

* *A Return to Love: Reflections on the Principles of "A Course in Miracles"* (HarperCollins, 1992).

"But I Should Be . . ."

Hope is dangerous. Dreaming of a bigger life means opening myself up to the possibility of disappointment. In my world, whenever I fantasize about trying something new, worries like "*What if I fail?*" linger in my mind. If I don't catch myself giving in to apprehension could scare me from *ever* trying anything new.

I've spent most of my life wrapped in fat like bubble wrap, carefully insulating myself from the outside world. Nothing hurts when you're hiding in sweatpants. Staying at home on the couch seemed safer than following any dream I had. Taking unnecessary risks was something I historically tried to sidestep. I could fall flat on my face! Plus, taking chances meant I'd have to show the world who I really was. That might not be pretty. The armor (and the sweatpants) would have to come off. *Um, no thanks.*

Gambling on a dream forces you to reveal your underbelly. There is a chance no one will like what I have to say, or worse, they might laugh or ridicule my foolish attempts at bettering myself. Rather than venturing out into a very judgmental world, I have a history of choosing to stay at home. Netflix does not judge. I can binge-watch episodes with a bowl of popcorn in my lap and avoid all that nonsense—*right*?

What surprises me, though, is how this never works. Even when I'm trying to hide in my living room, deep down I *still* can't let myself off the hook. In between episodes, I feel an itch to turn off the television and DO SOMETHING. *Do anything but watch TV!* I hear a nagging voice URGING me to make a different choice. Instead of starting the next episode, I think:

"I should be reading. I should be at the gym. I should be making dinner."

I should be, I should be, I should be . . . (You fill in the blank.)

(No way! You hear that voice, too?)

None of us REALLY wants to watch Netflix until we die. Deep down, we all want more out of life. Everyone has a dream. If not because of the after-school specials we grew up with, then because Oprah said we should: "What would I do if I weren't afraid of making a mistake, feeling rejected, looking foolish, or being alone."*

If you could pick anything in the world and *you knew you would be successful at it*, what would you choose to do?

For me, my answer has always been the same. I didn't want to learn Italian or how to dance the tango. My dream has always been *to get my spiraling weight under control.* I wanted to achieve what Oprah also struggled to do—*I dreamed of fixing my weight problem.*

The problem with aiming toward such a high goal is that *it's likely to be hard.* That might seem obvious and make you laugh, but for some reason we all think losing weight is supposed to be easy. Oprah, with a personal staff of chefs and physical trainers, still hasn't figured this out completely. What makes me think I'll be able to?

For so long, I failed at every attempt to change my eat-

---

* *What I Know for Sure,* by Oprah Winfrey (Flatiron Books, 2014).

ing habits. I would lose a little weight at first, hear compliments and encouragement from family and friends, but then sabotage myself (or give up) once I hit a roadblock. After many boomerang attempts at weight loss, it almost seemed easier to keep further attempts secret or not try at all. Surely everyone was laughing at me behind my back, right? I feared people didn't want to say anything about my weight loss because *they didn't expect it to last*. Deep down, I admit I probably agreed with them. Every time I went on a diet, I felt like a ticking time bomb. Everyone around me seemed to be holding their breath, waiting for my diet to blow up. I suspected that's why some of my friends would pretend *not to notice* I had lost weight.

There is a skill most of us lack when it comes to weight loss: it's NOT counting carbs or calories; it's getting back up after falling down.

Trying to "diet" inevitably leads to making mistakes. That's to be expected. The problem is that *we don't know what to do when that happens*. We feel like failures and lose all hope. Sadly, we think we have to be 100 percent perfect all the time. Then, because we don't know how to recover after screwing up, which is completely normal, most of us *just give up*.

We need to practice resiliency. We need to learn how to bounce back when things get really hard. Resiliency doesn't come naturally in the weight-loss arena—it's just too emotional of an issue. For this reason, I recommend you develop this life skill *outside the realm of weight loss.*

Learn how to step into a place *where you feel scared,* where you don't know what the outcome of your actions will be, and push forward anyway. Some call this experience blind faith (others say it's stupidity!), but I think there is value in taking risks to better yourself. By *embracing vulnerability,* we gain strength and confidence. This certainly will feel weird and uncomfortable at first! If (and when) something goes wrong, however, you'll learn how to face the challenge and stand up tall again. *This is how you build resiliency.*

For me, I feel most vulnerable when putting myself in a position of being **criticized, laughed at, or rejected.** This looks or sounds different to everybody, so here are examples of when I personally feel defenseless. Can you relate to any of these? All of these situations drum up the same inner feelings for me. Albeit at varying levels, in every one of these situations, I feel queasy, scared, and hesitant. I am filled with self-doubt, and my inner voice tries to protect me by telling me to STOP. It's so much safer to just PIPE DOWN and avoid these high-risk situations entirely, rather than face disappointment or complete failure.

I Feel Exposed When I'm . . .

- Seeing my loose skin (*and there is a lot!*)
- Stepping on the scale
- Getting undressed, even when I'm alone
- Going to the doctor
- Walking into the gym (*Every. Single. Time.*)

- Walking into a fitting room
- Receiving medical-test results
- Asking for help
- Going on a job interview
- Wearing a bikini (or any swimsuit, really!)
- Asking for feedback
- Saying, "I love you"
- Volunteering to go first
- Dancing or singing in front of others
- Making romantic gestures
- Wearing bright colors
- Honestly sharing my feelings
- Not knowing the answer
- Connecting with others
- Trying to look sexy
- Wishing for more
- Starting something unfamiliar
- Failing at something
- Initiating physical contact
- Going on a first date
- Admitting I'm wrong
- Wearing fitted clothes
- Asking for a promotion or a raise
- Receiving a work evaluation
- Trying something new
- Reading reviews of my writing

By putting myself in these vulnerable positions, I sometimes fall right on my face. The boots I thought were so fabulous at the store might cause a snicker from my teenage children. The doctor might give me suspicious results from my mammogram. I may not get the promotion at work I was hoping for. The point is, I put myself in situations where I was uneasy and I didn't know the outcome. Sometimes things go your way, but other times, luck is not on your side. Learning how to overcome disappointment or failure helps develop the valuable skill of resiliency. Your ego learns it can recover. All is not lost. You will become more confident in the ability to recuperate when things don't go your way.

Learning how to stand up again after a fall directly translates to helping you lose weight. When things don't go your way, you'll need to draw upon skills of resiliency to try again. Believe it or not, overcoming challenges becomes easier. You gain more confidence in your ability to conquer anything!

10

WHERE IS THE FINISH LINE?

Maintenance Starts the First Day, Not the Last

While visiting my ninety-nine-year-old grandmother in the hospital over Thanksgiving, I could see her frail, skeletal body was shutting down from infection. Rather than enjoy her favorite whipped cream–topped pumpkin pie, she pushed away the tray in disgust. *In my family, we don't turn away desserts. That's when I knew it was serious.* Despite the severity of her illness, Grandma pulled on the sleeve of my plus-sized sweatshirt and bragged, *"Stephie, I weigh a hundred pounds. Can you believe it?"* Her eyes twinkled with joy. Grandma spent her final moments celebrating a return to high school weight.

I shouldn't be surprised at my grandmother's obsession with size. She projected her own inadequacies onto me for my entire life. My childhood memories of my grandmother are littered with critical statements masked as polite "concern"

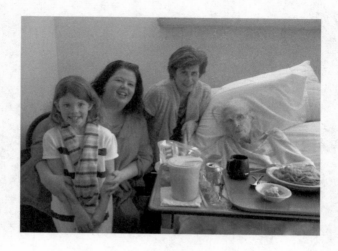

over the way I looked. While her intentions might have been pure, what I heard was an underlying message: *"You aren't good enough."*

Grandma's insecurities about herself were contagious. Without knowing why, I felt embarrassed about my size throughout elementary school. I learned to be ashamed of my height and weight, knowing I looked different than the other kids did. I was placed on various diets and dragged to community aerobics classes starting in second grade. *Girls go on diets,* was the message I heard, *because they need to be fixed.*

One Christmas, my grandmother surprised me with a cassette-tape Walkman. (Yes, I'm *that* old!) Though muffled by the sound of John Mellencamp in my earphones, I overheard my grandmother making snide comments to my mother that she hoped the Walkman would "motivate Stephie to exercise and lose that baby weight." I felt crushed and embarrassed by her comments. I immediately resented that Walkman.

I was nine when this happened, but I clearly remember her saying those words, some thirty-five years later.

The recorded messages we hear inside our heads are not our own thoughts. They are the opinions of our family, our partners, or even from the media. These messages are not the truth. What we *actually* think or feel about ourselves is replaced by all of this noise.

For decades, I heard my grandmother's voice and not my own: *"You are too big, too pudgy, and you eat too much."* I felt unworthy. I felt different from the other kids. I was someone who needed fixing. Her disapproval replayed in my heart so often that I became convinced it was all true. I was *told* I had a weight problem; therefore, I *must* have a weight problem. I expected myself to be overweight.

This self-fulfilling prophecy worsened with age. I became the stereotypical jolly fat kid who avoided playing sports, ate too much junk food, and rebelled against anything "healthy." I avoided exercise at all costs. I spent free time on the couch, watching movies. I was drawn to sedentary hobbies like drawing or writing, *not* playing outside.

While I point to my childhood memories to make a point here, I also take responsibility for my own decisions. As an adult, my size continued to grow. From high school to college and beyond, my weight climbed steadily. If I was a traded stock, I'd be compared to that of Apple. There was nothing but growth; I was a blue chip, baby! By the time 2006 rolled around, I was at my heaviest. I was closing in on a new decade in age, married, and desperately trying to juggle the responsibilities of raising two small children while working full-time. The Great Recession of 2007 to 2009 hit my family hard. Like a lot of our neighbors, our home was facing foreclosure. *I had a lot going on.* I coped with the stress in the only way I knew how: I ate. My weight inched toward three hundred pounds, the threshold mark at which household scales stop working. I remember going in for an annual physical and reading my chart when the doctor stepped out of the room. I read "Morbid Obesity, Class III" scrawled under my stats. I didn't even know that was a thing. Did that mean I was dying?

Even when I started having success losing weight with DIRTY, LAZY, KETO, I was afraid to go back to the doctor. I was terrified someone would refer to that diagnosis—again. I wanted to lose as much weight as possible to avoid being placed in that awful BMI category. With only changes in my food selections, I was able to lose fifty pounds or so pretty easily. But then one day it seemed to just sloooooooow down. DIRTY, LAZY, KETO worked for me until it didn't. Don't laugh, but it was a very sad day when I had to admit to myself that eating habits alone might actually have limitations for weight loss! Before the stall, I was convinced I wouldn't ever have to exercise. So far, the weight had come off pretty easily without breaking a sweat! I started questioning that theory, though, when my rate of losing weight changed from losing ten pounds a month to just a few measly pounds. (*That sounds so annoying in retrospect, I know!*) Perhaps I knew in my heart that I needed to exercise to break the plateau, but getting started sure wasn't easy.

You might laugh, but it took weeks to get off the couch. I'm *that* stubborn.

"Exercise? You don't need no stinkin' exercise!" my brain fought back. What would I do, anyway? I didn't know how to do any sports, and I *definitely* didn't belong to a gym. *When* would I even have time to exercise? There was not enough time in the day in my already packed schedule. I worked full-time and had two little kids and a husband to take care of. And, *I already felt so overwhelmed.*

A friend suggested putting exercise on the calendar—a whole *month* from then. What? That didn't make any sense.

"Like a dentist appointment?" I asked.

"Yes," she encouraged. "Circle a random date on the calendar and write, 'Go for a walk.'"

"Hmmm . . ." That sounded harmless enough.

I took her harmless advice and flipped the page on my calendar, scrawling "E-DAY" on an arbitrary future date.

Believe it or not, the anticipation of that walk taunted me every time I noticed it on the kitchen calendar. The details of *how* to exercise baffled me. *What* would I wear? *When* would I shower? Do people put makeup on *before* or *after* exercising? *Where* would I even walk? Now, looking back, I think how absurd that all sounds.

I don't think it was actually the logistics that caused so much anxiety. The darker truth is that I was afraid of being laughed at. My family, my neighbors, strangers driving by— would they make fun of the big lady waddling down to the mailbox, huffing and puffing, out of breath? Furthermore, the volume of my grandmother's critical voice played louder than ever in my head. I worried that exercise would be pointless because my weight loss had already stopped. It would be a waste of time, right? With my low self-esteem I feared I'd gain my lost weight back anyway, *just like before.*

By the time that day on the calendar entry came around, I was prepared (at least on paper). I made arrangements for the kids to carpool to school so I could get a head start on my day. There would be plenty of time for showering later! I pulled up my 4X Danskin fleece jogging pants and laced up "old school" leather tennis shoes found in the garage. I might have looked ridiculous, but guess what? I went out for a walk anyway! *Elvis had left the building.* Joggers passing me gave me a nod, neighbors "tooted" their horns while driving by, and dog walkers briskly chimed a quick "Mornin'." No one laughed at me (because no one cared!). There was no snickering or pointing of fingers. I faced my fear and survived the walk. Then the funniest thing happened—I started to cry.

I cried, you see, because I was having fun. This shocked and surprised me. I was enjoying myself! I started to cry because I couldn't believe I'd wasted so much time trying to convince myself to get off the couch.

In actuality, it wasn't just weeks I wasted anticipating that calendar entry, it was more like thirteen years. Somehow, with raising a family and developing a career, I had prioritized myself last. It took that single walk to provide perspective.

I started walking regularly. Within a short amount of time, I progressed from quickly walking to include bursts of jogging within the walk. At first, I could only run the length of a tennis court before becoming winded. Despite thinking I was going to die, I challenged myself to jog a little farther each time I tried to run. I would pick a tree or lamppost in front of me and focus on running only to that point. The steps started adding up. Running very far didn't happen overnight, mind you. *Let's not get ahead of ourselves!* While I wasn't a fast or conditioned runner, I was a consistent one. I kept at the walking (and bits of running) almost religiously. I committed to Monday, Wednesday, and Friday. *I never missed a day.*

The pounds started coming off again. By adding just this little bit of exercise to compliment DIRTY, LAZY, KETO, I was losing weight again at a steady pace. I surprised myself one day by running a full mile *without stopping*! This was the first time in my entire life (grade school included) that I had run a full mile, and I was pushing forty, people! That watershed moment unleashed something I didn't know I had inside of me. Soon, running one mile became two, then a 5K, and on to much, much more.

Out of all the runs I've completed since then, my proudest moment occurred when my daughter saw me run for the first time. She was in fifth grade (ironically, about the same age as me when I received my Walkman). We were on a spontaneous trip to the neighborhood park, her on a bike, me on foot. She started pulling ahead, so naturally, I broke into a slow jog to catch up. She saw what was happening and abruptly stopped pedaling.

"MOMMY IS RUNNING!" my daughter screamed at no one in particular. Her reddened and confused face stared at me with wide eyes. Whether she was afraid for my life, in shock, or feeling utter joy, I couldn't tell, but the moment was priceless.

In all of her years of being alive, my little girl had *never* seen her mommy run. *As in ever.* It was at this moment that I realized I wanted to change the kind of parent I was for my children. I didn't want to be one of those moms who sat on the couch all day barking orders from a seated position, never playing with their kids. I'm well aware of the research that shows overweight parents are likely to raise overweight children. Being overweight is miserable. My daughter deserved more!

I became even more motivated to push myself. I wrote a new script to play inside my head, but this time in my own voice. I deleted the demeaning and judgmental tape loop from my childhood and replaced how I talked to myself with inspirational phrases. The words I chose were positive, kind, and supportive: *I can do this. I am stronger than I realize. I am a runner.*

My growing confidence helped me reach outside my comfort zone. I registered for upcoming races, a 5K, 10K, and then a half marathon. The weirdest thing happened as I conquered short-term goals in front of me: instead of stopping, I yearned for more challenges. Shockingly, I kept raising the bar even higher. Even though I was afraid, I wanted to see *just how far I could go.* Little did I know, *striving for more is a common human experience* (especially among healthy people!). It's natural to want to push the limit of our physical capability. The way I felt after exercising was addictive. I had never felt more powerful, capable, and beautiful, *all at once.* I wanted more.

Within two years of "slogging" my way around the neighborhood, I worked myself up to the distance of a marathon, which, unbeknownst to me, was a whopping 26.2 miles.

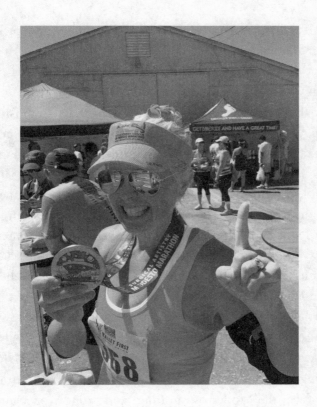

In 2005, despite all odds, this forty-year-old (former Miss Couch Potato) finished the Modesto Marathon in first place. Yes, you read that correctly—*first place*!

I had read that the Modesto Marathon offered an Athena Division as a competitive racing opportunity. Just like in wrestling competitions, there are weight divisions for running. Athenas, like the grand horses they are, represent the heavyweight division. If a larger runner was brave enough to qualify to compete, they would first have to publicly weigh in at the marathon expo. Taking place in a city conference center, a marathon expo is an opportunity for runners to mingle with dozens (sometimes hundreds) of vendors and pick up race materials.

For some reason, the ridiculous concept of competing as a heavyweight appealed to me. Maybe I could win a prize! I saw this as my once-in-a-lifetime opportunity to finish first (*or maybe at all!*) in an athletic competition. I would be celebrated, not criticized, for being a larger athlete; that kind of praise rarely happens.

So let's stop for a moment. I want you to picture the girl who once hid her seat belt from the flight attendant with an in-flight blanket, pretending to be asleep because the seat belt wouldn't buckle and was too embarrassed to ask for an extender. This is the same girl who told the hostess at her favorite Mexican restaurant that she would prefer "that table over there" (and not the booth they were walking toward) because she could eyeball *not fitting* in the booth.

I want you to picture that girl—*YES, THAT GIRL*—making the spontaneous decision to walk up to the racing director at the Modesto Marathon and proudly proclaim, "I want to compete in the Athena Division. I eagerly volunteer to be weighed on a huge scale in front of everyone at this convention center!"

Can you imagine the humiliation? Further, what if I couldn't follow through? Seeing how this was my first marathon, I wasn't sure I would finish the race itself, let alone run faster than the other Athenas. Clearly, in signing up for this added level of competition, I had lost my marbles.

This is what exercise does to you. It gives you ridiculous confidence in ways that losing weight never could. When you experience the small joys of being able to walk up a flight of stairs without becoming out of breath, you are eager to take on more. Obviously, change doesn't happen in one fell swoop. Transforming yourself into picture-perfect health doesn't mean signing up for a year at the gym or committing to a summer boot-camp program; your health improves by *consistently* making teeny, tiny decisions, the ones that don't seem to matter, day in, day out.

When you combine physical activity, no matter how advanced, with a newly scripted, encouraging voice inside your head, the possibilities are endless!

With practice and repetition, exercise and healthy decision-making build up to become a permanent lifestyle.

One of the greatest ironies of healthy living is that it takes constant emotional effort (at least for me, anyway); I have to continually work at it. The "old me" often tries to creep back into my thoughts. When I recognize that pesky voice, I swat at it like a fly. When she whispers for me to take the elevator, park closer, or sleep in, I smack back with my sassiest tone: *No, thank you; I'm getting my steps in.*

It's not always that easy, though, I'll admit. That alluring, seductive voice can be convincing; she knows exactly how to push my buttons. For example, even two years later (in 2017), when I arrived at the convention center to pick up my bib for the New York City Marathon, I stopped at the entrance, becoming almost paralyzed with fear.

"You don't belong here," I heard inside my head. "Look

at the amazing athletes around you. *You are NOT one of them!"*

Despite being a sponsored runner from PowerBar (*that's right!*), I felt completely inadequate, embarrassed, and fraudulent. I felt I didn't belong in the VIP wing with the elite athletes. *PowerBar had made a mistake inviting me to New York City! Maybe I should just go back to the airport.* I sounded like Eeyore from Winnie the Pooh.

Instead of mentally preparing for the 26.2 miles ahead of me, I battled inner demons trying to rip apart my confidence. How sad that I couldn't fully enjoy a once-in-a-lifetime experience.

Everyone shows up to a marathon with some nervousness, true, but not everyone shares my history. I may have lost over a hundred pounds on the outside, but on the inside, I'm still the same person. I've realized as the stakes increase with stressful situations, my anxiety skyrockets to unprecedented levels. I have a long history of freaking out instead of facing my fear.

Competing in marathons has helped me anticipate and prepare for emotional turbulence. By expecting waves of self-doubt, I'm not caught off guard as often. Training for a big race is just like preparing for a speaking engagement or taking on a hefty project at work. It's normal to feel anxiety about uncertainty. The struggle is learning how to muddle through without hurting myself. Instead of mollifying my anxiety by eating unhealthy foods, I've realized that showing some compassion is much more effective.

In the past, when faced with tense situations, I only had one coping strategy: to eat. High-sugar, high-carbohydrate snacks provided me with immediate relief. A hit of Gummy Bears left

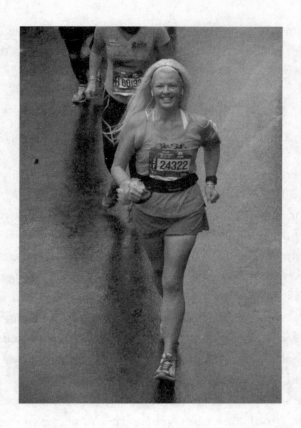

me feeling calm. Shoving popcorn in my mouth, fistfuls at a time, lowered my blood pressure. I would eat so fast and furiously that the snack would be over and I'd be dumbfounded as to where it all went. I wouldn't even have a memory of eating the snack! I've spent my entire life turning to food to handle almost every emotion, and changing that behavior will not, *I repeat, not,* happen overnight. So how can you handle this instead?

I've learned to become more self-aware during times of pressure. Maintaining my weight loss hinges upon the many innocuous decisions I make to handle stress. I ask for help when I need it. I talk things out if needed. I plan for the worst, hope for the best, and don't let myself become overconfident.

Be Selfish: Give from the Saucer, Not from the Cup

Every Friday night when I was growing up, my family went out to dinner at Bob's Big Boy. Leftover cash from our "envelope" money-management system funded this weekly treat. Even though we had the money set aside for the restaurant, my mom never splurged. She silently watched everyone order whatever they wanted from the menu. When it was her turn, however, Mom told the waitress to bring an order of scrambled eggs, the cheapest thing on the menu. By scrimping on her order, she ensured we would have enough cash to pay the bill. That's how I was raised. Sacrifice. Put the family's needs first and your needs last.

I repeated this same pattern when I became a wife and mother. I took care of everyone else's needs before tending to my own. I thought that was expected in my role. I did the family's laundry, cleaned the house, cooked dinner, and even packed individual suitcases for vacations. Truth be told, it never crossed my mind to do things any other way. When my kids were little, I scoffed at the idea of having a babysitter. My husband and I never "went out," as I didn't think anyone could possibly watch my children as well as I could. I judged other moms who dropped off their little ones (even for an hour) while at the gym exercising. I didn't need anyone's help, I believed. I would do everything myself.

When my husband lost his job and our income was drastically reduced, my children were not affected in the least. They still went to private swim lessons, wore name-brand shoes, and ate Happy Meals. I, on the other hand, cut back on everything. I dyed my hair in the kitchen sink rather than go to the salon. I painted my own nails. When the hem of my work pants wore thin, I used Super Glue (and even a stapler, if I'm being totally honest) to keep the edges from fraying, continuing to wear them to work rather than buy something new.

I cut corners in every direction to keep our household running, but mostly from my own needs. That came with a high cost, though. By taking care of everyone else first, I was left feeling exhausted. I doubt anyone in my family noticed my sacrifices, because I did it all voluntarily with a closed-lipped smile, not uttering a single complaint. No one knew how I was feeling inside. I wish I could fess up to feeling resentful during this time of my life, but I don't actually think that was the case. Like any martyr, I relished the importance of my role. I was the cement that held us all together.

Instead of talking about feeling overwhelmed, I managed my worries in the most rudimentary way: I ate. I avoided lingering concerns about calories and hid the scale toward the back of the linen closet. I ate junk food and found solace in the drive-thru. I had pizza delivered to my house. It wasn't pretty, but I survived that dark financial period of my life by eating my way through it.

When I started to change what I ate (and subsequently lose weight), other parts of my personality were forced to evolve, too. I realized the meal on my plate was just one small part of a larger picture. I would need to morph the domestic role I held in my family if I was going to make any progress. *Just because I was a wife and mother didn't mean I didn't exist, too.* My own needs, independent of my family's, had to be equally recognized as important. The old me would have called that behavior selfish, but today I call it absolutely critical. If there is nothing else you take away from this book, remember this: **your needs matter.**

While it's clichéd to tell a woman to "put on her oxygen mask before helping children," putting yourself first is a necessary step for you to take before you can successfully lose weight. Unfortunately, most women are like me and have trouble following these directions. It's instinctual for women to take care of other people first. Making self-centered choices could invite judgment, mostly from other women. We fear being called a bitch, or worse, a bad mother.

Here's a thought to entertain, though: *"SO WHAT?"* Let people judge you. Let them call you names. Would that really be so terrible? I used to think putting my needs first would make me a bad mother. I've come to realize that the opposite is true. **I've become a better parent for taking care of myself first.**

#BreakTheRules

When you start to assert your needs at home, be prepared for a potential backlash. Your family might resist. I remember when I asked my elementary school–aged kids to pack their own suitcases for a trip so Mommy could go for a morning walk—*they completely freaked out!* You would've thought I'd asked them to clean toilets, they were so appalled! This story is so funny to me now, as my kids have grown into teenagers who wouldn't DREAM of letting me pick out their clothes! Back then, however, turning over the simple task of packing a suitcase caused a lot of heartache. I'm a "control freak," for sure, so it was hard for me to let go of deciding what the kids would be wearing on vacation. In my heart, I knew packing for trips made me feel overwhelmed. I realized that delegating this responsibility would really help me relax. Yes, the children's packed clothes might not match, or a toothbrush might get forgotten, but on the flip side, I could start a vacation feeling more centered. Trying to take care of myself before others made a world of difference, even though the transition was hard.

I still hate asking for help. I like to pretend I can "do it all." At least now, though, I'm aware that "doing it all" comes with a price.

Putting yourself first means accepting that others will do things differently than you would. It's not helpful to delegate a task to free up some "me time," but then hover and criticize about how the job is executed by someone else. I remember when my husband took over the role of taking the kids to school in the morning so I could run. I needed to leave the house earlier to be able to exercise, shower, and then get to work on time, and taking the kids to school didn't allow for that full routine to happen. Of course, there had to be some fallout. About a month into our new schedule, my daughter brought home her school pictures. I noticed right away she had the most beautiful smile. Then something strange jumped out at me: *she was wearing pajamas!* I had to let go of my attempts to be a perfect parent. I couldn't do it all. I needed to take care of myself first and then do the best I could for everyone else. Letting go, and having a sense of humor about things, helped make the transition smoother.

Evidence of consistent commitment to my health happened this week with my running. According to the Nike app on my phone (which records every mile that I run), I reached

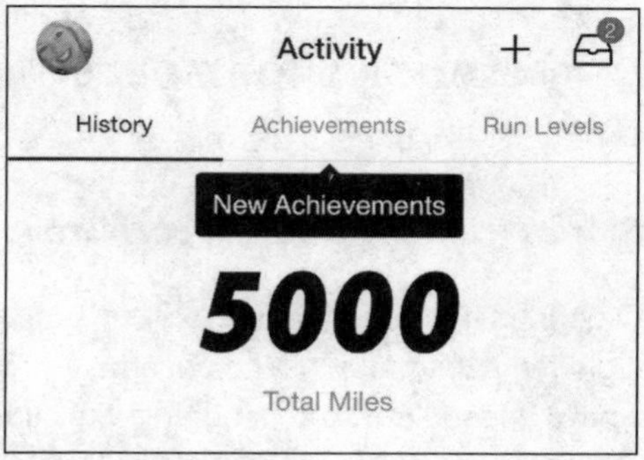
Activity
History
Achievements
Run Levels
New Achievements
5000
Total Miles

a new milestone. I surpassed running more than five thousand miles. FIVE THOUSAND MILES since I started running back in 2013! I accomplished this unbelievable distance by putting on my running shoes over nine hundred individual times. Had I freaked out over the pajamas in my daughter's school photo, or had I never asked for help to begin with, this unthinkable milestone would not be happening.

Be selfish, my friends. Put yourself first—I dare you!

Imagine what extraordinary things *you* will be able to do.

To Infinity and Beyond! Results Beyond Weight Loss

In addition to weight loss, DIRTY, LAZY, KETO provides so many other health benefits, most of which have yet to be fully explained or explored by science. By eating higher fat, moderate protein, and lower carbohydrate foods, I've observed that my own body has experienced less inflammation.

Weird, huh?

Apparently, DIRTY, LAZY, KETO foods are less irritating to the body.

After years of suffering from obesity and chronic headaches, I was desperate for a change. My energy levels were at an all-time low, and I began every morning by chasing coffee with Diet Coke and Tylenol. Even though I weighed close to three hundred pounds, it didn't click that the foods I ate might be contributing to my chronic daily headache and overall lack of energy. I reached for every migraine medication on the market and even sought out specialists for treatment. Pills and shots couldn't make the problem go away for very long; medication only masked the symptoms for a short period of time. The headaches *always came back*.

I accidentally discovered the benefits of eating anti-inflammatory foods. I initially followed DIRTY, LAZY, KETO just to lose weight, but I soon experienced additional benefits. Once I became fat adapted, my energy levels soared and the crippling headaches STOPPED. The irony is not lost here. The sugars and starches I previously depended on for quick energy boosts ended up being the culprit for my feeling tired and dull. Once I eliminated these foods and replaced them with low-carbohydrate vegetables and fruits, quality proteins, and healthy fats, the positive effects were immediate. Mental clarity, sustainable "even" energy, and pain-free temples were the most notable physical effects I experienced.

Looking back, I realize that whenever I ate sugary or high-carb foods, I experienced a chain reaction of events that would spin me out of control. After enjoying the brief rush from eating the starch and having my blood sugar spike, the good feeling would end abruptly. My skin felt clammy, my stomach swelled, and my mind felt fuzzy. I would progressively become so tired that I needed to close my eyes. The only relief I could find to reverse my symptoms was to eat MORE carbs again; what a vicious cycle!

Because of this realization, I advocate being consistent with the DIRTY, LAZY, KETO lifestyle and avoid reintroducing starchy or sugary foods back into your routine. Seemingly innocent "vacations from healthy eating" promote rampant inflammation throughout the body and rev up the sugar addiction cycle *all over again*. The times when I ignored my own advice and gobbled down French fries, I felt GREAT for about five seconds. Almost immediately, the tide turned and regret set in. I became bloated and sweaty. A painful headache soon developed, and I usually experienced gastrointestinal distress (*that's a classy way to say I was full of gas*). Agreed, French fries taste amazing, but they make me feel absolutely terrible after eating them, both emotionally and physically, just moments later! *So. Not. Worth. It.*

By no means am I perfect. Temptations will always be a challenge. When I find myself thinking I might be able to handle eating a so-called treat, I've learned to stop and try to think it through. Weight loss or maintaining my weight isn't always the most convincing reason to stay away from high-carb foods. For me, I have to think about the other benefits DIRTY, LAZY, KETO has provided. Changing my perspective to help me overcome temptation is effective not only for me, but for many people. **Focusing on outcomes other than weight loss might just be the most powerful tool you have for keeping the weight off long-term.**

#BreakTheRules

You don't have to just take my word for it. Let's hear what others have to say from my Facebook support group. I have to warn you, though: every time I read these comments I start to cry. When I started this journey, I just wanted to drink beer and eat chicken at a barbecue, remember? I had no idea just how powerful my story would become. DIRTY, LAZY, KETO may have started off as a guide for weight loss, but it quickly became so much more to thousands upon thousands of people. DIRTY, LAZY, KETO is not a diet, *it's a way of life.*

FACEBOOK SHOUT-OUT

Benefits Beyond Weight Loss

Comments from the DLK Support Group

"I have ENERGY!" —Robin

"My diabetes 2 is reversed. My doctor is telling everyone about me!" —Junior

"No more headaches. I used to get migraines regularly, *but not anymore.*" —Kim

"Sex Drive A+." —Anonymous

"I can walk normally for the first time in decades. I don't have joint pain." —Jackie

"I have a clear face. *No more acne!* I've even started dating." —Tonya

"I don't get heartburn like I used to. I even stopped keeping Tums in the car." —Gary

"No more blood-sugar meds. I have normal triglyceride levels and my blood pressure is normal. I almost can't believe it. I started this to lose weight, but this is even better." —Connie

"I sleep like a baby." —MC

"I feel more confident and have great self-esteem now." —Ramona

"The awful bloating? *Gone.*" —Jess

"Mental clarity. I feel much more focused at school." —Alicia

"I don't have sleep apnea anymore. My wife is so happy!" —Ray

"Mentally, I feel very positive." —Dana

"My HBA1C is officially out of the prediabetic range." —Linda

"I can practically run up the stairs. I used to gasp for air, so this is a really big deal for me." —Lanette

"My confidence has awoken!" —Roberta

"I don't have to use my inhaler anymore." —Jordan

"No more acid reflux." —Tanya

"I have normal blood pressure now. NO MORE medication." —Ed

"I'm not walking around hungry. The cravings I used to feel have stopped." —Nic

"It's like I never had arthritis. I wish I had known about this years ago. The pain is gone." —Ruth

"I don't need to use insulin." —Cyrus

"Everything is just 'better' . . . physically *and* emotionally." —Maribel

"The rosacea on my face is almost invisible." —Patricia

"Normal bloodwork all around!" —Johnathan

"*Finally*, no more snoring." —CJ

"My knees don't hurt anymore." —April

"Diabetes is in remission!" —Travis

"The swelling in my legs stopped." —Keith

"I was told I have 'pep in my step' now." —Jiu

"My son hasn't had a seizure since we started this." —Meghan

"I'm awake! No more naps or falling asleep when I watch TV." —Elijah

"The tremors in my hands? Well, they don't happen now." —Betty

"IBS is gone after having it for fifteen years." —Tyler

"I'm PREGNANT! I'm so thankful this helped my Polycystic Ovarian Syndrome." —Stacey

The Big Picture

These days, when I buckle my seat belt on an airplane, I have the biggest smile on my face. *Seat belts that fit NEVER get old!* I buy fancy bras now at Victoria's Secret, *because I can.* Want to go to an amusement park? Yes, LET'S GO! I'm not worried about going over the weight limit or not fitting inside a ride anymore. **My weight or attitude doesn't hold me back. I feel like I'm finally living the life I was meant to live.**

People often ask me what the hardest part of losing 140 pounds was. You might guess running a marathon. *(I have finished twelve of them, thank you very much.)* Or was it "coming back" after having body parts and a tumor surgically removed? (Nope, that wasn't it, either, though that REALLY sucked!)

I'll tell you what the hardest part was: saying no to buttered popcorn at the movies, and learning to say yes to me. Yep, my answer is that simple— and yet complicated at the same time.

I discovered it's the little things that actually matter. **The tiny, day-to-day decisions (that don't seem like a big deal) are really what's most important to make this work.**

Over time, being consistent (but not perfect) about self-advocacy adds up to a lifestyle change; that, my friends, is what DIRTY, LAZY, KETO is all about. It's so much more than food!

Living according to this bit of advice (*oh,* and eating VEGETABLES!) is my personal secret sauce for making DIRTY, LAZY, KETO a sustainable lifestyle. *Now you know!*

At this point, dear reader, I hope you are fired up to choose the bigger life. Armed with a DIRTY, LAZY, KETO shopping list and a strong-willed, sassy attitude, you are now prepared to enter battle. I have given you all of my tools. You know all of my secrets. You are ready to begin your own journey to become the best YOU!

Like in any war, there will be combat. Victory tastes sweeter when you have to overcome great challenges. Don't be afraid of obstacles. You have the tools to handle them. When things get rough, I want you to remember:

- You are *not* alone. We are all struggling.
- Be *selfish*. Put your needs first.
- *Choose* your choices. Be honest with yourself about potential consequences.
- It's the *little* decisions that matter. They really do add up to something big!

The scale will become your best friend some days, worthy of "onederland" happy tears and Instagram photos. You, too, will dance inside fitting rooms after trying on smaller sized clothes. There will be unexpected private moments that take your breath away, like the first time you wrap a bath towel *fully around* your naked body. All of a sudden, you can rise from a chair without using your arms. Your new shape will fit comfortably in airplane bathrooms and be able to walk straight through narrow aisles. Even getting in and out of a pool will be easy! Losing excess weight will unburden you. There is no telling what's in store for your future! I expect your weight change will only be a small part of your butterfly transformation. Through the DIRTY, LAZY, KETO lifestyle, you will gain *so much more*.

You can do this, my friend! Join me in the regular-size section of department stores. Join me in the "normal" BMI category. Become part of the 1 percent that keeps their weight off—*for good*! I know you will be successful. Please share your progress photos with me (*well, maybe not the towel pictures*). I can already envision your before-and-after selfie tagged with #dirtylazyketo.

If I can lose half of my entire body weight and maintain the weight loss for more than seven years, I'm betting with all of my heart that you can do this, too.

You don't have to be perfect to be successful. Go ahead, my friend,

#BreakTheRules!

#KetoOn!

Stephanie

XXOO

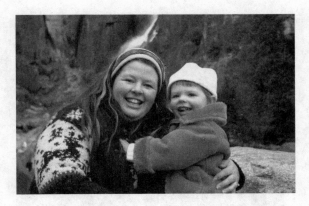

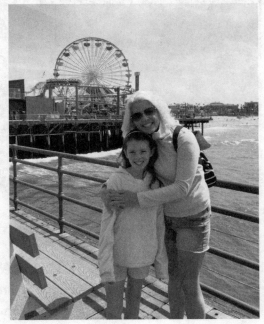

The fondest memory of my weight-loss journey was the day my elementary school–aged daughter wrapped her arms around me and yelled in surprise, "Mommy, my arms can reach completely around you!"

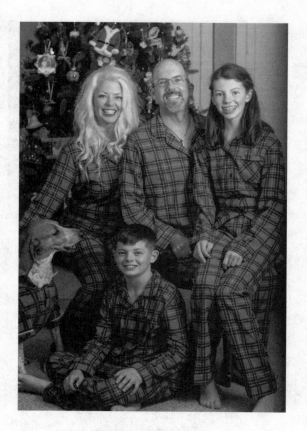

Testimonials

"Living this 'dirty, lazy' ketogenic lifestyle has helped me personally to not only lose one hundred pounds but to keep it off after years of yo-yo dieting and two failed attempts to lose weight through major surgeries. Stephanie's books are all that you need to get started and guide you along every step of the way as you get closer and closer to realizing your own goals and potential!"

"[Stephanie] makes the diet easy to follow. She also has a great sense of humor. Loved this book."

"This book made total sense to me. Easy. Just-give-me-the-facts kind of read. I'm twenty pounds down in sixty days, but more important, I feel great."

"This book was great. The thing that sets this book apart from other books is how REAL the author is. She's very transparent and reiterates throughout the book that it's just a guide and does not implement shame in any way. She gives great tips and helps you feel as though you won't fail if YOU hold yourself accountable and use common sense."

"I love the book. I thought she was witty and informative. I like that I can still have my glass of wine on this diet."

"It clears the air in keto land. . . . It's simple to read, a very sensible approach without all the hype! After reading the book, you realize everything you need to succeed is at your local grocery store . . . no gimmicks . . . and that's what I love about it."

"It was great! She absolutely knows my struggle!"

"A fresh, REAL life-changing approach to the ketogenic way of eating by someone who has done it. Stephanie is brave enough to share ALL of her journey with us, not just the victories."

"A fine blueprint filled with down-to-earth advice and guilt-free life experiences for us all. A practical and inspiring book."

"The book is amazing! Really helpful and in language that is easy to understand!"

"Easy to read; gets you started right away. Very well written, funny."

"Easy read and so relatable. Stephanie is a breath of fresh air. I look forward to moving ahead with this program and making it my own."

"It helped me become more comfortable eating what I like versus a strict diet. I was feeling guilty about my daily Diet Coke. Not now."

"Easy to read and friendly. No judgment, and isn't that what it's all about?"

"I followed it lazily and dirty! I, too, was amazed how easy it was!!"

"Easy to read, real, relatable, encouraging, fun . . . fast paced."

"Great book with a realistic approach! Loved reading it, and loved the humor!"

"This was an easy read with great advice and humor to go with it. It's a real book for real people who want to lose weight!"

"It's a real person's approach. I could relate. It makes sense and didn't come across like a 'do-or-die' plan. Common sense and natural humor!"

"This is the best book I've read on keto. Explains things so simply. I can understand exactly how to do this and why!"

"Extremely helpful for those just starting out trying to grasp this way of eating. . . . I wish I would have known about it a year ago when I first started trying on and off to eat this way."

"It was funny and informative; I couldn't put it down until I read the whole thing."

"Best keto book out there!! I've spent weeks going to bookstores, looking through keto books. This one feels like she is talking to me in my language!!! I'm just starting this journey, and I now feel like I can actually do it!!"

"Finally, someone who can explain keto in a simple, easy-to-understand way of eating."

"I will stay with DIRTY, LAZY, KETO for the rest of my life, since in five months it has led me to get off insulin after twenty-five years of injecting myself."

"DIRTY, LAZY, KETO changed my life. I went from being a pancreatic-cancer survivor with onset diabetes 2 from the pancreas surgery to completely changing my diet based on this book. Now my blood sugar is in control. . . . Age fifty-five and I've never felt younger in my life."

"Thanks to DIRTY, LAZY, KETO . . . for the first time in my entire life, I now actually enjoy shopping for clothes and eating healthy!"

"I no longer need blood pressure meds. I can tie my shoes without getting out of breath. I'm down countless inches and forty-two pounds! I still have about thirty-five pounds to lose, but I'm finally happy in my skin! DIRTY, LAZY, KETO boosted my confidence and saved my life."

"There is nothing that I miss. My energy level is so awesome. I do not need to take a nap. My inflammation is gone, my arthritis has improved 100 percent. I've finally gotten below 170, lost several inches; I feel great and I look good—healthy and strong. I think most diets deprive us, and that is why people give them up. But DIRTY, LAZY, KETO doesn't deprive me."

"At seventy diagnosed with stage 3 cancer of the uterus. Had complete hysterectomy, chemo, radiation and chemo. I was at 212 pounds. Started keto because sugar feeds cancer. EVERY test and checkup is great since. And to top it off I have lost 51 pounds in seven months."

"Stephanie is like the coach/friend/sister/drinking buddy I've always wanted—talking the way she talks, helping with the things I really need, and completely real with advice."

"I've never seen such fantastic results in my life. . . . I don't feel dragged down anymore, and my energy level has gone up. . . . DIRTY, LAZY, KETO is my life now, and I couldn't be happier!"

"I learned it's okay not to be perfect. I can still do this my way and lose weight and be healthier."

"I have been overweight since I was pregnant with my first child—forty-three years ago! This is for me. No cravings and I'm not starving all the time. I'm tired of all the diet police and feeling down on myself. I've got grandkids to enjoy."

"Still truckin' along here with DIRTY, LAZY, KETO. . . . Down seventy pounds since October, insulin dosage one-third of where I started, metformin no longer needed, and no more thyroid medication! Cholesterol and triglycerides in great ranges. This really works!"

"*DIRTY, LAZY, KETO* arrived two days ago, and all my chores were put on hold because my entire day was spent curled up with the book. I couldn't put it down. I understand so much more about this new lifestyle! I'm on my way now."

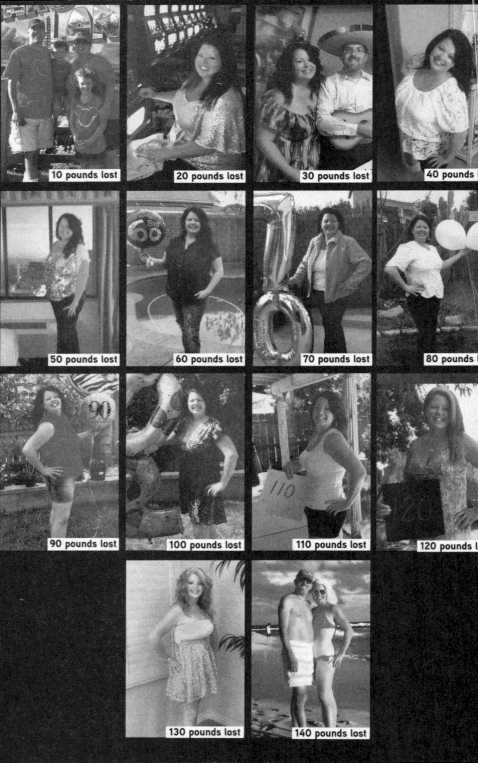

10 pounds lost

20 pounds lost

30 pounds lost

40 pounds lost

50 pounds lost

60 pounds lost

70 pounds lost

80 pounds lost

90 pounds lost

100 pounds lost

110 pounds lost

120 pounds lost

130 pounds lost

140 pounds lost

INDEX

carbohydrates (carbs) (*continued*)
   LCHF (low-carbohydrate, high-fat)
      diet, 23–24
   minimum number of, 51
   net, 24, 33, 40–41, 48, 50–52, 90,
      155, 226–28
   saving for later, 58
   slow-burning, 21–22, 39
   see also sugar
celery vs. coffee creamer, 38–39
chaffle, 22
cheating, 185, 303–4
   intentional eating vs., 190–94
   rationalization of, 190–91
   rethinking, 218
cheese, 100–101
cheese waffle (chaffle), 22
cholesterol, 110–11
chocolate cravings, 169–70
   recipes for, 172–74
circle of trust, 274–75
clothes, 134, 139–42, 144–47
cocktails, 84–86
coconut milk, 60
coffee, 61, 58
   bulletproof, 58–62
coffee creamer vs. celery, 38–39
comfort foods, 164, 295
comments:
   from friends and family, 268–83
   from strangers, 311–12
compliments, 268–83
confidence and self-esteem, 51,
      193–94, 307, 311, 317, 318–20,
      326, 336
cravings, 168–70
   for chocolate, 169–70
   for fried and fattening foods, 168,
      170–71, 172, 175–77

recipes for, 172–77
   for sweets, 69, 157, 168–69,
      172–74
cream, 60, 99
criticisms, 268–83

dairy alternatives, 98–99
dairy products:
   cheese, 100–101
   cream, 60, 99
   in Dirty, Lazy, Keto food pyramid,
      49, 91, 97–101
   grocery list for, 234–36
   milk, 98–99
   yogurt, 97–98
dehydration, 23, 194, 196
desserts, 69–76, 110, 157, 160,
      161
   high-carb, 46
destructive coping mechanisms,
      293–95
destructive internal dialogue,
      313–14
detoxing, 183
diabetes, 16, 37, 198
diets, 117–18, 149–50, 323
   Atkins, xvi, xxiii–xxiv
   LCHF (low-carbohydrate, high-fat),
      23–24
   myths about, 152–56
   reasons people stop, 119–21
dinner, 62–66
Dirty, Lazy, Keto, 7–55
   day-to-day management of,
      283–85; *see also* environment
   defined, 17–18
   differences between other keto
      diets and, 53
   "dirty" in, 9, 18, 19

ABOUT THE AUTHOR

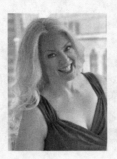

Stephanie Laska, M.Ed doesn't just talk the talk, she walks the walk. She is one of the few keto authors who has successfully lost half of her body weight (140 pounds!) and maintained that weight loss for seven years and counting. Her sass and honest approach to the keto diet has been shared on *NBC's Today Show* and in *Reader's Digest, Playboy, First for Women Magazine, Costco Connection Magazine,* and *Yahoo News.* As the author of *DIRTY, LAZY, KETO*, Stephanie Laska's story and image are celebrated in media outlets such as *Muscle and Fitness: Hers*, Daily Burn, the San Francisco Marathon, the Big Sur International Marathon Race Guide, RunDisney, and even in a Groupon!